The Longterm Care of the Coronary Patient

Risteard Mulcahy MD FRCP FRCPI FFCM
Late Director of Cardiac Department and of Cardiac Rehabilitation and Secondary Prevention Clinic, St. Vincent's Hospital

and

Professor of Preventive Cardiology (Emeritus), St. Vincent's Hospital and University College, Dublin, Ireland.

Published with the aid of an educational grant from Parke-Davis.

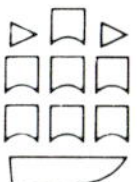

CHURCHILL LIVINGSTONE
EDINBURGH LONDON MELBOURNE AND NEW YORK 1990

CHURCHILL LIVINGSTONE
Medical Division of Longman Group UK Limited

Distributed in the United States of America by
Churchill Livingstone Inc., 1560 Broadway, New York,
NY 10036, and by associated companies, branches
and representatives throughout the world.

First published 1991

ISBN 0-443-04673-5

Printed in Great Britain by Bell and Bain Ltd., Glasgow

Preface

This monograph is based on our experience in the cardiac rehabilitation and secondary prevention clinic established at St. Vincent's Hospital in 1966. The St. Vincent's programme was designed to provide a cost effective rehabilitation service for patients with coronary heart disease and for post-operative patients with valve disease. It was also designed to provide longterm assessment of factors determining the prognosis of patients surviving myocardial infarction.

Implicit in the service was the routine involvement of all members of the medical and paramedical cardiology staff in rehabilitation and secondary prevention counselling, and the provision of a service which would require no major extra facilities in terms of staff, equipment, space or expenditure. The service was designed to suit any large district or teaching hospital.

Some aspects of current cardiac rehabilitation are based on empirical or rational grounds rather than proven evidence derived from valid and adequate trials. Hence, some doubts or even controversy are inseparable from some of the recommendations we make. It is not my intention to provide an extensive list of references when dealing with aspects of rehabilitation which remain the subject of controversy, because of the need to avoid listing selective references which might give a biased view of such issues. Instead, I have provided a list of papers, editorials, and reviews which I believe give a balanced and comprehensive overview of these uncertain issues.

This monograph was written during a sabbatical visit at the Austin Hospital in Melbourne. I am most grateful for the hospitality and support which I received from Dr. Alan Goble, Dr. Marion Worcester and Elaine Race. I thank my daughter-in-law Caroline Mulcahy for her careful and expert preparation of the manuscript, and Carol Kennedy and Michael Martin for assistance with the preparation of references.

I wish to acknowledge financial assistance from the British and Irish Heart Foundations, the Leverhume Trust, the European Social Fund, The Medical Research Council of Ireland and various corporate and personal supporters.

Ireland, 1990 R.M.

Acknowledgements

I am grateful to many colleagues who have worked with me during the past 30 years since the Cardiac Department at St. Vincent's Hospital was first established and when our interest in coronary heart disease causation, prevention and rehabilitation commenced. In particular I owe special thanks to Professor Noel Hickey, Dr. Ian Graham, Vivien Reid, Dr. Leslie Daly, Carol Kennedy, Denise Comerford, Ronan Conroy and Nancy Grogan.

Both Valerie Feehan and Una Leydon, sisters successively in charge of coronary care, played a major role in the success of our rehabilitation programme. The Hospital authorities were at all times supportive. Philomena Moriarty and her staff at the Computer Department of University College, Dublin provided invaluable and rarely acknowledged assistance. Nurses and resident doctors, too numerous to mention, also deserve my gratitude.

Contents

SECTION 1

Introduction

1. The current status of cardiac rehabilitation

The longterm care of the coronary patient, including rehabilitation, is an aspect of cardiology which has evoked too little interest among the majority of cardiologists and physicians. It has generally been divorced from the activities and interests of the clinical cardiologist, preoccupied as he is with the diagnostic and therapeutic techniques which have shown such spectacular advances in recent years. It is implicit in current attitudes that rehabilitation does not require the personal attention of the cardiologist or the physician dealing with heart disease. When the facilities are available, we assume that it can be well enough attended to by other personnel, such as the occupational therapist, dietitian, social worker, physiotherapist and psychologist. In the cardiological world today, it can be said that the rehabilitation of patients with coronary heart disease and other chronic cardiac conditions receives too little attention because cardiologists see themselves as being exclusively concerned with diagnostic and therapeutic activities.

Another serious deficiency, particularly in longterm cardiac rehabilitation, has been the very limited participation of general practitioners and community physicians, a circumstance which one might attribute to a failure of communication between the hospital cardiologist and the community doctor. This monograph is particularly designed to advise general practitioners and community physicians about the principles of cardiac rehabilitation.

The neglect of cardiac rehabilitation is evident in all western countries, including those with a high incidence of coronary heart disease. Australia is a suitable country to quote because it has an established and developed economy with medical services comparable to other developed nations. National data based on Australian rehabilitation practices are available from the National Heart Foundation in Australia (Worcester 1988).

Of the 153 eligible hospitals studied, only 26 provided out-patient group exercise programmes and 36 provided group educational programmes. Medical and psychological counselling was haphazard and provided by only a small minority, apart from advice the patient may have received from the physician. The utilisation of the services of physiotherapists, dietitians, and occupational therapists left much to be desired. It was concluded that, in many hospitals, there was poor co-ordination of rehabilitation services and there was generally a negative attitude to rehabilitation measures. The author concludes that the emphasis on life-saving measures and intervention, such as drugs and surgery, had not been matched by considerations of the patients' longterm needs and that the cost benefits of rehabilitation were not appreciated.

WHY LONGTERM CARE?

It is precisely because rehabilitation after myocardial infarction and heart surgery is an essential component of good cardiological practice, needing the full attention and encouragement of the cardiologist, that this monograph has been written. It is because many doctors tend to ignore the fact that most forms of heart disease, including coronary heart disease, are chronic conditions requiring not only intervention to treat acute events and complications, but also advice and management to slow down and stop the progress of the underlying disease, to reduce subsequent morbidity and premature mortality, and to ensure a return to a normal good quality life. It is now readily apparent that good rehabilitation practice confers important physical, psychological, social and personal benefits on our patients. However, such practices are only available to a minority of our patients. Too often patients are discharged from hospital after a myocardial infarction, or after coronary or valve surgery, and are not given the guidelines and support to enable them to return to a normal life in professional, social and physical terms. While active interventions, including surgery, angioplasty and drug requirements, are invariably part of our therapeutic recommendations, the identification and elimination of risk factors are neglected to the detriment of the patient's recovery, subsequent progress and quality of life.

The object of this monograph is to provide the necessary guidelines to ensure that patients who survive an acute cardiac episode, such as an infarction, or who have had heart surgery, are given an optimum opportunity of returning to a normal life and of enjoying a reduced risk of delayed complications, of further coronary events or sudden death. These guidelines can be provided without adding significantly to the cost of medical care in terms of facilities, equipment, and personnel. Successful rehabilitation and secondary prevention measures can be provided for the large number of patients who are in need of such services, but effective and widespread application of rehabilitation will only be achieved by a lead from the cardiologist and hospital physician in co-operation with other rehabilitation personnel. Without such co-operation from physicians and surgeons, and from the family physician, good longterm management of patients with coronary and valvular disease is not easily achieved.

The role of the cardiologist

The failure of most cardiologists to interest themselves in longterm care is the primary cause of poor rehabilitation practices. Limitations are based on a number of factors, the most important being our preoccupation with acute exacerbations and complications, and our neglect of the chronic underlying process of disease. Other factors, too, contribute to our shortcomings. These include the tenuous communication which exists between our hospitals and the community, the general practitioner's limited commitment to health promotion and prevention, and his isolation from hospital and hospital colleagues. They also include the failure to employ other health personnel in management, both during the acute illness and subsequently, and our haphazard attempts to educate the patient and the patient's family, and to involve them in longterm management.

Cardiac rehabilitation defined

How are we to define cardiac rehabilitation? It is the process whereby we return patients to as normal a life as possible in personal, social, psychological and medical terms. It must be based on future objectives, and it may require prolonged supervision by the family doctor or physician. It will almost certainly require some lifestyle changes to improve function and quality of life, and to reduce complications and the progression of the underlying disease. In concept, cardiac rehabilitation is no different from the management of diabetes, rheumatoid arthritis, hypertension and other chronic conditions and, like these conditions, it requires the full co-operation of physician and hospital staff, family doctor, patient and family. It should be unacceptable in this time of great achievements in cardiology that patients are returned home after a heart attack or after heart surgery without ensuring that they and the family are properly informed about subsequent care and secondary preventive measures. It is also unacceptable that, although we are aware that sustained compliance with treatment measures and lifestyle changes is less than satisfactory, and that it requires repeated encouragement and reinforcement of advice, we do little to ensure that such compliance is maintained.

What type of rehabilitation programmes are available? The situation varies, from the majority of hospitals and physicians who pay little or no attention to rehabilitation, to the provision of elaborate and expensive institutional programmes. The latter programmes are relatively few, are mostly found in Middle and Eastern European countries, where they may be freely available to every patient, or have been established because of the special clinical or research interest of a physician or group of physicians. Effective rehabilitation programmes vary in their design and complexity, from the simple out-patient advisory services providing secondary prevention advice (including risk factor intervention and home-based exercise programmes) to the highly elaborate in-patient institutional programmes. All programmes have advantages and possible drawbacks, which shall be discussed later. At this juncture, suffice it to say that effective cardiac rehabilitation can be achieved without the more complex institutional type of intervention. The complexity and cost of these programmes are such as to be prohibitive for the great majority of patients and to all except the most affluent countries.

We need to provide a service which is applicable to all patients, irrespective of their economic circumstances and the nature of the health delivery system, and to all hospitals, whatever their size and budgets. An efficient and cost effective rehabilitation service can be organised within the normal in-patient and out-patient activities of a hospital, and may require only the established staff and equipment which are normally part of the clinical cardiology services (Hickey & Mulcahy 1985, Bethell 1988).

HISTORY OF CARDIAC REHABILITATION

Modern cardiac rehabilitation had its origins in the 1950s when isolated physicians began to question the old conservative notions about the management of heart disease, an approach based on prolonged hospitalisation and immobilisation, cautious and prolonged convalescence, and an emphasis on the need for permanent restrictive physical, social and vocational measures. Early research was largely directed at evaluating the hazards of returning to work and the possible consequences of physical exercise. The ability of the damaged heart to respond to physical training was also a source of interest and investigation.

Now we are satisfied that return to work is not only safe for the great majority of patients, but that it is desirable from the psychological and quality of life points of view. We are satisfied that physical exercise, particularly of the aerobic type, is not only safe if properly prescribed and complied with, but that it is also desirable and may contribute directly or indirectly to reducing subsequent morbidity and mortality (Oldridge et al 1988). We are also satisfied that the scarred heart, the damaged heart, and the heart disturbed in other ways, is capable of responding to an appropriate exercise programme by improving its physiological work capacity in line with improved pulmonary function and peripheral mechanisms (Sebrechts et al 1986).

Modern concepts of rehabilitation

Great progress has been made in the past 25 years in stabilising the rationale and the efficacy of exercise programmes, of returning patients to a normal professional life, and of reducing the misapprehensions and anxieties associated with diseases of the heart. The objectives of cardiac rehabilitation in 1989 are now broad-based, thanks to the progress made in earlier years, and include social, physical and sexual activities. To encourage an improved quality of life, more attention is being paid to adverse psychological changes associated with heart disease, including anxiety, depression, loss of confidence and denial, and personality traits, such as type A behaviour.

Modern cardiac rehabilitation also places strong emphasis on risk factor identification and elimination, and on the behaviourial changes required to slow down or stop the atherosclerotic process or to encourage regression.

The value of cardiac rehabilitation in restoring patients to their rightful place in the social and family structure, and in improving prognosis and beneficially affecting the adverse psychological effects of a heart attack, has been firmly established. However, we are still faced with the reality and the challenge that this knowledge is poorly and unevenly applied to the great majority of patients who suffer a heart attack. It is also poorly applied to those who suffer from chronic angina of effort, those who have had heart surgery or those who suffer from valvular or other less common cardiac conditions. The challenge still remains to encourage physicians and general practitioners, and particularly cardiologists, who can so effectively give a lead, to incorporate rehabilitation and longterm secondary prevention in their clinical work.

Comprehensive cardiac rehabilitation must be based on reasonable evidence of efficacy, on feasibility in relation to the patient's capabilities, circumstances, inclinations and wishes, and on safety and acceptability from the medical, social and cultural viewpoints. Ideally, judgement of efficacy and cost benefit should rest on the best possible evidence, such as the properly designed randomised controlled trial. However, many of the recommendations we make in the course of orthodox cardiac rehabilitation programmes have not or cannot be shown to be of incontrovertible benefit because of logistic and other difficulties in carrying out suitable trials (Greenland & Chu 1988). We are therefore dependent on less reliable but nevertheless strong circumstantial and intuitive evidence to justify many of our recommendations.

Good rehabilitation is basically good doctoring and, like good doctoring, is as inseparable from art and human judgement as from science. Good doctoring cannot always be measured by p-values. If we measure the cost of intervention in terms of inconvenience, risk and expenditure against the perceived benefits, we should help rather than harm our patients. In expressing opinions about rehabilitation, I am conscious of the deficiencies in our knowledge but I am motivated by the rationale of our recommendations and by long experience of our patients' response to our policies.

REFERENCES

Bethell H J 1988 How to set up a coronary rehabilitation programme. British Medical Journal 297:120-121

Greenland P, Chu J S 1988 Efficacy of cardiac rehabilitation services. With emphasis on patients after myocardial infarction. Annals of Internal Medicine 109:671-673

Hickey N, Mulcahy R 1985 Cardiac rehabilitation program: St Vincent's Hospital rehabilitation programme. Journal of Cardiac Rehabilitation 5:386-388

Oldridge N B, Guyatt G H, Fischer M E, Rimm A A 1988 Cardiac rehabilitation after myocardial infarction. Combined experience of randomized clinical trials. Journal of the American Medical Association 260:945-950

Sebrechts C, Klein J L, Ahnve S, Froelicher V F, Ashburn W L 1986 Myocardial perfusion changes following one year of exercise training assessed by thallium-201 circumferential count profiles. American Heart Journal 112:1217-1226

Worcester M 1986 Cardiac rehabilitation programme in Australian Hospitals. National Heart Foundation of Australia, Canberra

FURTHER READING

Konig K, Denolin H, Dorossiev D (eds) 2nd edition 1983 Myocardial Infarction. How to prevent, How to Rehabilitate: Scientific Council on Rehabilitation of Cardiac Patients, International Society and Federation of Cardiology, Boehringer Mannheim

Sobel B E (ed) 1989 Bibliography of the current world literature: ischaemic heart disease. Current Opinion in Cardiology 4:569-623

Wenger N K (ed) 1986 The Education of the Patient With Cardiac Disease in the Twenty-First Century. Le Jacq Publishing, New York

VIDEO

Your life in your hands: recovery from a heart attack 1990 The Coronary Prevention Group. London (20 mins).

2. Pathology and natural history

It would be inappropriate to discuss the pathology of atherosclerosis in great detail in this monograph but there are important aspects of its pathology and natural history which are helpful in understanding the approach to treatment and to rehabilitation. While atherosclerosis is a widespread system disease of arteries, it does have a well recognised predilection for certain vessels and certain vascular systems. The coronary arteries, the aorta and its main branches, particularly to the head and neck, and certain leg vessels are prone to manifest the disease. The distal vessels of the arm, the internal iliac, the profunda femoris, and other vessels are relatively immune to atherosclerosis for reasons which are not clear.

Large vessels tend to be affected more than the smaller ones, a fortunate circumstance for the by-pass surgeon. The disease tends to be patchy rather than diffuse, and plaques are likely to occur at certain locations in the vessels where hydraulic stresses may lead to increased endothelial permeability and thus to the vulnerability of the arterial intima (Say 1972). Locations just beyond sub-divisions are particularly vulnerable as are segments of arteries where there are abrupt curvatures or angles, or where there may be narrowing with post-stenotic turbulence. Loss of laminar flow, turbulence and alterations in flow rates may be important factors in determining the site of atherosclerotic plaques, and the propensity to atheroma may be increased by a higher pressure than normal within the vessels. Hence, the pulmonary artery, not normally prone to atherosclerosis, may show plaques in patients with pulmonary hypertension, and the various grafts used to by-pass vessels are also prone to atherosclerotic changes.

The coronary angiographer is familiar with the patchy nature of atheroma. Critical lesions tend to occur at the origins of the three main vessels, at or beyond sites of primary branches, and less commonly in the left main stem. Proximal changes in the marginal branches of the circumflex, and the diagonal branches of the anterior descending and the right coronary artery are common.

In less than 5% of patients with clinically documented myocardial infarction, no significant lesions may be found in the coronary vessels on angiography. These unusual cases may be attributed to arterial spasm, revascularisation of an acute thrombus, embolism or other non-coronary causes (Castello et al 1990). The majority of symptomatic patients show a greater or lesser degree of involvement of the three vessels—the anterior descending, the right coronary and circumflex—while a smaller number show a dominant left main stem lesion, or single or two vessel disease. Rarely, extensive ectatic changes may be evident in one or more of the vessels. This presents as a 'rosary beads' appearance which can be quite striking in severe cases, with alternating aneurysmal and constricted segments. We do not know what determines the diffuse or patchy nature of the disease, but there is some relationship between morphology and the patients' age, risk profile, and possibly ethnic origin. Jews are more prone to ectatic disease, young patients with isolated risk factors, such as heavy cigarette smokers or young women on the anovular pill, tend to have isolated discrete lesions. Older patients and those with severe hyperlipidaemia are more prone to diffuse involvement of the three vessels. These are by no means hard and fast rules, but these findings are sufficiently common to be factors which will influence our judgement in the management of patients. A knowledge of the distribution, severity, extent, and nature of the coronary lesions is important because the coronary morphology is an established factor in determining longterm prognosis, although not as important as left ventricular function. Coronary morphology is an important guide to management, particularly when surgery or angioplasty are therapeutic options.

PROGRESSION AND REGRESSION OF ATHEROSCLEROSIS

There is still much to be learned about the factors which determine progression and regression of atherosclerosis. Clinical and pathological data confirm experimental evidence that the progress of the disease may be rapid and may be measured in months rather than years. The presence of advanced and extensive disease in young people with homozygous and heterozygous hyperlipidaemia provides such evidence, as did the autopsy findings in young American soldiers who were killed in the Korean war. The very early onset of clinical coronary heart disease in homozygotes supports the view that rapid progress is related to the strength of risk factors to which the patient is exposed. As a corollary, it would seem logical that we should attempt to eliminate all identifiable risk factors if we are to retard progress of the disease in primary and secondary preventive practice.

There is substantial clinical evidence to suggest that progress of atherosclerosis may be retarded, arrested or reversed (Arntzenius et al 1985,

Blankenhorn et al 1978, Blankenhorn et al 1987, Blankenhorn et al 1988, Brensike et al 1984, Duffield et al 1983, Nash et al 1984, Nikkila et al 1984), evidence which is congruent with the results of experimental studies (Wissler & Vesselinovitch 1983). Those of us who have conducted long-term follow-up studies of patients with coronary heart disease will have seen patients who remain well and free from further symptomatic vascular disease for many years. In our follow-up study at St. Vincent's Hospital, of the 309 male survivors under 60 years seen with a first myocardial infarction between 1961 and 1969, 65 were still alive at the end of 1988 and 42 had had no further vascular episodes. There is limited evidence that longterm survival may be increased by elimination of risk factors in patients with established coronary disease and these results may be attributed to the retardation or non-progression of the underlying arterial process.

By advocating risk factor modification we may achieve non-progression or regression of the underlying arterial disease. We must be aware of the implications of such a concept.

What evidence have we of regression and under what circumstances does it occur? Evidence of regression has been found in the course of experimental angiographic studies (Nikkila et al 1984, Arntzenius et al 1985) and in animal models (Wissler & Vesselinovitch 1983). It also may be inferred from autopsy studies of patients who have died of carcinoma and other wasting conditions, where remarkably clear arteries have been noted in subjects drawn from a high risk population (Attman 1967). It is well established that a falling cholesterol level is an important and early marker of carcinoma and may be detected some years before the patient's death. These changes in cholesterol level are consistent with the findings of relative freedom from atherosclerosis and, in patients dying from carcinoma, strongly support the concept of regression.

There is accumulating evidence that regression may occur, but whether such regression can be attained to a significant or clinically important degree in patients with extensive, critical and advanced atheroma of the coronary and other vessels still remains to be proven. In advocating risk factor identification and control as an essential component of secondary prevention and rehabilitation, we are making reasonable assumptions about achieving probable retardation and possible regression of the atherosclerotic process, and therefore about an improvement in subsequent morbidity and mortality. We also may make assumptions about desirable modifications in platelet aggregation, free fatty acids, high density lipoprotein cholesterol levels, fibrinolysis, carboxyhaemoglobin, and other mechanisms affecting atherogenesis, thrombosis and arrhythmias, through smoking and dietary control, and exercise programmes.

The pathological basis of symptomatic disease

The presence of coronary atheroma does not necessarily imply the presence of coronary heart disease. Many subjects found to have significant and even advanced coronary atheroma at autopsy will have been asymptomatic and unaware of their condition. The progress to symptomatic disease, whether it be sudden death, non-progressive angina, or myocardial infarction, is usually delayed until the arterial disease is advanced or until critical discrete lesions have formed. Hence most patients with coronary heart disease have advanced three vessel disease but there are many exceptions, where the condition may manifest itself clinically in patients with single or two vessel disease and, rarely, in those with little or no evidence of disease (Castello et al 1990).

From the pathological point of view, early symptoms may be associated with the gradual progress of atherosclerosis, but in most patients an acute underlying process superimposed on long-standing atheroma may lead to the gradual or, more often, the acute onset of symptoms. These include intravascular thrombosis, rupture or dissection of an atherosclerotic plaque, platelet aggregation and arterial spasm. The exact circumstance leading to an acute event is rarely apparent, although there is weak evidence that, in a few patients, climatic, seasonal, circadian, stress, exercise and life event factors may be implicated. The evidence of such behaviourial or environmental precipitating factors is not sufficiently strong or convincing to assist in providing guidelines for patients at risk, and generally recourse to such advice can be unnecessarily restrictive in retarding a return to a normal life. That is not to say that the important components of coronary rehabilitation, such as smoking control, appropriate dietary changes and exercise programmes, may not be useful in reducing the risk of thrombosis, platelet aggregation, and other adverse pathological processes.

Sudden death or acute myocardial infarction will be preceded by symptoms of unstable angina in more than 50% of cases. Unstable angina may present as recent onset or crescendo angina of effort, or with transient recurring rest pain. The mechanisms whereby the process progresses to infarction or life-threatening arrhythmias are poorly understood, but may be related to the various mechanisms associated with the onset of symptomatic disease, and alluded to above.

THE INFLUENCE OF RISK FACTORS ON MORPHOLOGY

We can attempt to identify subjects who are likely to suffer from atherosclerotic disease by studying their risk factor profiles. This subject is dealt with in greater detail later, but experience would suggest that the acknowledged coronary risk factors of hyperlipidaemia, hypertension and cigarette smoking tend to be differently associated with the location of atherosclerotic disease, as well as with the process in general. The specific association between cigarette smoking and peripheral vascular disease, between hypertension and atherosclerotic and haemorrhagic stroke, and between hyperlipidaemia and coronary artery disease is clinically apparent, although epidemiological, clinical and pathological data confirm that all three risk factors are significantly associated with atherosclerotic disease at all sites (Surgeon General 1979B). The specific associations alluded to above need corroboration by further studies, particularly as there are no plausible reasons why one risk factor may have a different morphological effect than another.

The widespread distribution of atherosclerosis in the body, and its concept as a systemic metabolic disease is confirmed, not only by findings at autopsy, but by the clinician who finds a higher than expected prevalence of combined stroke, peripheral vascular disease and other clinical manifestations of atherosclerosis in patients with coronary heart disease. The widespread nature of the disease confirms the importance of making every effort to slow down, stop or reverse the process of atherogenesis as part of our rehabilitation and management approach.

In considering the pathology and natural history of coronary heart disease, the clinician will also be concerned about the presence of other vascular and non-vascular conditions not infrequently found in coronary patients. Because cigarette smoking, hypertension, hyperlipidaemia, diabetes, and obesity cause multisystem disease, it is not surprising that patients admitted to coronary care are victims of more than one disease process. Peripheral vascular disease, transient ischaemic attacks, strokes, aneurysm, chronic lung disease, gout, diabetes, gall bladder disease—these are only some of the conditions which are not uncommonly found in coronary patients. This clustering of disease may play a major modifying role in management and in planning rehabilitation programmes.

REFERENCES

Arntzenius A C, Kromhout D, Borth J D et al 1985 Diet, lipoproteins and the progression of coronary atherosclerosis. The Leiden Intervention Trial. New England Journal of Medicine 312:805-811

Attman R F 1967 The curious interrelation between cancer and diseases of the arteries. Hospital (Rio) 72:1027-1053

Blankenhorn D H, Brooks S H, Selzer R H, Barndt R Jr 1978 The rate of atherosclerosis change during treatment of hyperlipoproteinaemia. Circulation 57:355-361

Blankenhorn D H, Nessim S A, Johnson R L, Sanmario M E, Azen S P, Cashin-Hemphill L 1987 Beneficial effects of combined colestipol-niacin therapy on coronary atherosclerosis and coronary venous bypass grafts. Journal of the American Medical Association 257:3233-3240

Blankenhorn D H, Johnson R L, El Zein H A, Vailas L I 1988 Dietary fat influences human coronary lesion formation. Circulation 78:89-96

Brensike J F, Levy R I, Kelsey S F et al 1984 Effects on therapy with cholestyramine on progression of coronary atherosclerosis: results of the NHLBI Type II Coronary Intervention Study. Circulation 69:313-324

Castello R, Alegria E, Merino A, Fidalgo M L, Martinez-Caro D 1990 The value of exercise testing in patients with coronary artery spasm. American Heart Journal 119:259-263

Duffield R G, Lewis B, Miller N E, Jamieson C W, Brunt J N, Colchester A C 1983 Treatment of hyperlipidaemia retards progression of symptomatic femoral atherosclerosis. A randomized controlled trial. Lancet 2:639-642

Nash D T, Gensini G, Esente P 1984 The progression of coronary atherosclerosis. Journal of Cardiac Rehabilitation 4:21-26

Nikkila E A, Viikinkoski P, Valle M, Frick M H 1984 Prevention of progression of coronary atherosclerosis by treatment of hyperlipidaemia: a seven year prospective angiographic study. British Medical Journal 289:220-223.

Say B L 1972 Localising factors in arteriosclerosis. In: Likoff W, Segall B L, Insull Jr. W (eds) Arteriosclerosis and Coronary Heart Disease. Grune and Stratten, New York.

Surgeon General's Report 1979B Healthy People. Report on health promotion and disease prevention. US Department of Health Education and Welfare, Public Health Service. DHEW publications 79-55071.

Wissler R W, Vesselinovitch D 1983 Combined effects of cholestyramine and probucal on regression of atherosclerosis in rhesus monkey aortas. Applied Pathology 1:89-96

3. Epidemiology and causation

Epidemiology has played a major part in advancing knowledge of the causes and prevention of coronary disease during the past 40 years. From early beginnings after the last great war, with the work of Ancel Keys and his colleagues in identifying hyperlipidaemia as the key risk factor (Keys et al 1966), and the start of the Framingham prospective study (Nash et al 1974), cardiovascular epidemiology has led the field in the study of the chronic diseases in populations. It has successfully identified the principal causes of atheroma and its clinical consequences, and, in association with parallel clinical, pathological, basic research, and animal studies, it has contributed substantially to the current rapid decline in the prevalence of coronary and total mortality in many western countries (World Health Organization 1989). The basis of our knowledge derived from cardiovascular epidemiological studies provides the rationale for the major intervention projects which are taking place in most western countries today.

Population and clinical studies of coronary heart disease causation have also played a major role in establishing the high standards of evaluation and of validation which are a feature of the modern epidemiological approach to the chronic, non-communicable disease of the latter part of the 20th century. It is likely that the coronary epidemic, which has swept the western world since the mid-century and which was common but not so readily recognised in earlier years, will no longer be a major public health problem in some western countries, at least during the more active years of life, by the end of the millennium. This view may hold good at least for those countries with active public health policies in the area of the chronic non-communicable diseases. The United States, Australia, and Finland have shown a dramatic reduction of between 35% and 50% in coronary mortality in the past 20 years. Figures 3.1a,b show the changes in coronary heart disease mortality which have taken place in various countries between the years 1969 and 1987 among men and women aged 30 to 69 years (World Health Organization 1989). These declines show no evidence of slowing. The decline in coronary mortality is following the equally dramatic fall in stroke mortality which has been evident for a longer time. The reduction is

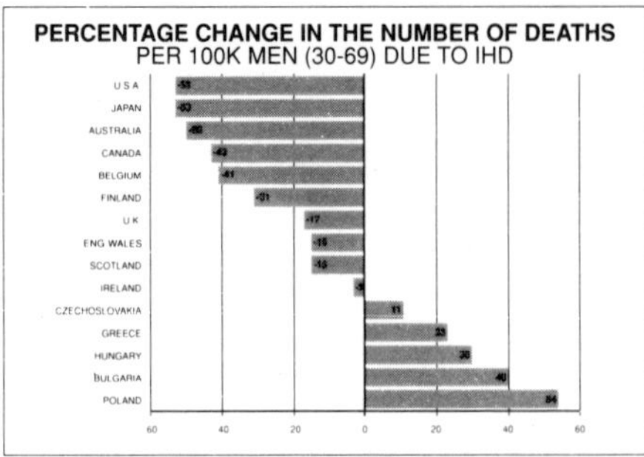

Fig. 3.1a Trends in coronary heart disease mortality in men aged 30-69 for various countries from 1969-1987.

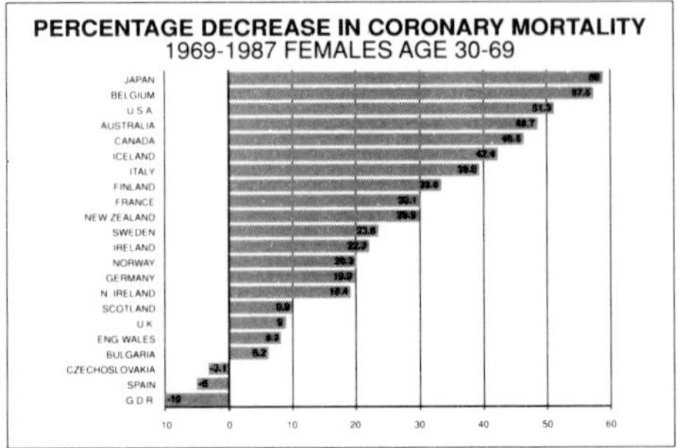

Fig. 3.1b Trends in coronary heart disease mortality in women aged 30-69 for various countries from 1969-1987.

particularly striking among the younger age groups and has led to a substantial improvement in life expectation in these countries.

The study of coronary heart disease was facilitated by the sensitivity and specificity of the diagnostic criteria. The presence of characteristic pain, with specific enzyme and ECG changes, made for the relatively easy recognition of the disease. This could not be said for stroke, with its different aetiologies, nor for other vascular conditions. The high prevalence of coronary heart disease, particularly in the younger age groups, made for easier epidemiological studies. However, the knowledge acquired about the aetiology of coronary disease has contributed to our knowledge of the causes and the natural history of stroke, peripheral vascular disease and aneurysm, and has identified the same risk factors—hyperlipidaemia, cigarette smoking and hypertension—as being important, to a greater or lesser extent, in their genesis.

THE RISK FACTOR CONCEPT

The knowledge of the causes and natural history of coronary heart disease derived from epidemiological studies has also contributed to our management of patients with established disease. While most cardiologists have been slow to apply this knowledge, there is increasing recognition that secondary prevention, through risk factor identification and modification, plays a vital role in the management and rehabilitation of patients with angina and in survivors of myocardial infarction. In my view, strict risk factor modification, combined with exercise programmes and guidelines aimed at improving quality of life, is the single most important component of rehabilitation and longterm management, at least in terms of reducing complications and improving prospects of event-free survival. One must acknowledge the contribution made by coronary artery surgery, angioplasty and drugs in reducing complications and in improving survival, but these are essentially palliative procedures while risk factor intervention has a plausible basis in retarding the progress of the underlying arterial lesions as well as reducing the impact and risk of other vascular and non-vascular conditions.

What is the evidence supporting the value of risk factor intervention as a component of longterm management and rehabilitation of the patient with coronary heart disease? It is based partly on the logic and plausibility of this approach, but there are some studies which would lend support to this management policy. The paucity of studies, particularly in relation to the control of hyperlipidaemia after myocardial infarction, can be attributed to the difficulties in designing such studies. These include the confounding influence of other therapeutic modalities, and the need for multi-centre studies to provide sufficient numbers and end-points, with all the problems of cost and variations in standards of diagnosis, management and end-point assessment associated with multi-centre trials.

Cigarette smoking

The clearest evidence of benefit comes from studies of smoking cessation after myocardial infarction (Mulcahy 1983). Most published studies show a longterm benefit in terms of subsequent mortality of 25-50% in those initial smokers who stop compared to those who continue. A few studies confirm a reduction in subsequent non-fatal infarction, and a study from my own research group of the influence of subsequent smoking in post-infarction angina of effort showed a significant reduction in its prevalence during the first six years after the initial attack (Daly et al 1985). There are other major benefits following cessation of smoking, particularly in the prevention of stroke, peripheral vascular disease, lung cancer and in the amelioration of chronic lung disease, which makes this a mandatory step in management.

Hyperlipidaemia and hypertension

There is less clear-cut evidence in relation to the control of hyperlipidaemia as a component of secondary prevention. All dietary studies aimed at elucidating the value of hyperlipidaemia control have had serious deficiencies in design, mostly related to inadequate numbers studied and to insufficient length of follow-up. Of the nine studies reported, four showed no benefit and five showed reduced morbidity or mortality in the intervention groups (Ball et al 1964, Bierenbaum et al 1970, Hansen et al 1962, Kallio et al 1979, Leren 1970, Medical Research Council 1968, Morrison 1960, Phillips et al 1988, Rose et al 1965). No study reported adverse effects of dietary control. However, the Coronary Drug Trial of the secondary prevention of coronary disease reported improved survival after 12 years in patients treated with nicotinic acid compared to controls (Canner et al 1986). In our experience, compliance with dietary advice aimed at control of hyperlipidaemia can be achieved without great inconvenience to the patient and the family, subject to the provision of proper guidelines and to occasional supervision by the dietitian.

There is still inadequate evidence relating to the benefits or adverse effects of hypertension control in secondary prevention. Few studies have been reported, probably because hypertension control is ethically indicated in view of the incontrovertible evidence from primary prevention studies that such control is beneficial in preventing stroke, left ventricular and renal failure. It would be difficult to provide a control group under such circumstances. The gradual fall in hypertensive morbidity and mortality in the past 50 years or more testifies to the benefits of the modern therapeutic approach, without accounting for other, largely unexplained, factors which have been operative before widespread drug and non-pharmacological methods were adopted.

In a limited non-randomised trial we reported an adverse prognosis in hypertensive survivors of myocardial infarction who were deemed to have been inadequately treated subsequently, compared to normotensive and adequately treated hypertensive survivors (Graham et al 1978). Connolly et al (1983) also reported improved survival in treated compared to untreated hypertensive patients with coronary disease. It is significant that a number of primary prevention trials showed benefit in treated patients in terms of stroke, left ventricular failure and renal failure, but not in patients with coronary heart disease (Multiple Risk Factor Intervention Trial 1982). This apparently anomalous result has been attributed to the adverse effect of certain hypotensive drugs on the lipid profile of patients, suggesting that the potential beneficial effects of blood pressure control by these drugs is lost by their adverse effect on the lipid profile. While the benefits of hypertension control in the secondary prevention of coronary heart disease remains speculative, and may never be elucidated, there is no evidence that control of moderate or severe hypertension can have an adverse effect. This, and the likelihood of preventing other hypertensive complications, underlines the need for blood pressure control in the long-term management of the coronary patient.

Hamalainen and her colleagues from Finland reported on the effects of multiple risk factor intervention in coronary patients (Hamalainen et al 1989). They showed that, in patients subjected to smoking and hypertension control, and to dietary modification of hyperlipidaemia, total coronary mortality and sudden death were significantly lower over a 10-year period compared to controls not subjected to secondary preventive measures.

Exercise

The influence of exercise programmes on subsequent morbidity and mortality has been widely studied. There are inherent problems in such studies which make assessment of the independent influence of exercise very difficult. While most reported studies confirm non-significant benefits of regular aerobic exercise and the feasibility of achieving a training effect in coronary survivors, it is virtually impossible to separate a possible independent effect of exercise from the other behaviourial and life style modifications which are so often associated with exercise and which may also influence subsequent prognosis. Nor is it easy in these trials to allow for the large number of patients who fail to comply with the prescribed exercise, and for the control patients who are 'contaminated' by the current consensus in favour of greater activity after a heart attack. Metanalysis of 14 comparable randomised exercise studies confirms that patients subjected to post-infarction exercise and secondary prevention programmes have a mean reduction of 25% in subsequent coronary mortality compared to subjects not included in such programmes (Oldridge et al 1988).

It is now established that appropriate aerobic exercise, regularly carried out over the longterm, is safe in patients who are properly evaluated before the exercise programme is prescribed. There is no need for anything more than a moderate training effect. There is clear evidence that regular exercise, if incorporated into the patient's life as an enjoyable or useful activity, can be continued indefinitely and is likely to improve quality of life and compliance with other desirable life style changes.

Other risk factors

Other risk factors for coronary heart disease include diabetes mellitus, obesity, stress and type A behaviour. However, unlike hyperlipidaemia, hypertension and cigarette smoking, they have not been shown to be causative and their control for the specific purpose of the secondary prevention of coronary disease cannot be unequivocally justified. However, their control is necessary if only to prevent complications specific to diabetes and obesity, and to improve the quality of life and the motivation of those subject to abnormal stress or showing features of type A personality behaviour.

Epidemiological studies, in association with clinical, pathological, basic research and animal studies, confirm the role of hyperlipidaemia, hypertension and cigarette smoking as the three major independent causative risk factors in high risk populations. Studies of populations with low mean cholesterol levels, a low prevalence of hyperlipidaemia, and a low fat content in the national diet, confirm that they have a low incidence of coronary heart disease. Japan and Korea are two such countries, although the Japanese people are heavy smokers and are particularly prone to hypertension. It is likely that hyperlipidaemia is the key to the genesis of atheroma and coronary heart disease, and that hypertension and smoking become important risk factors only in populations with a high incidence of hyperlipidaemia.

It is generally postulated that other unrecognised metabolic or environmental risk factors may exist, mainly because the above mentioned factors, whether deemed to be causative or not, fail to account for the totality of cases in clinical and population studies, when employing logistic regression and other statistical techniques. For example, educational and social class are determinants of coronary heart disease risk (Mulcahy et al 1984, Rose & Marmot 1981, Buring et al 1987). The less privileged members of society in the United Kingdom, Ireland and the United States are at higher risk of coronary heart disease because of an unfavourable profile, particularly in relation to smoking, alcohol, hyperlipidaemia and hypertension. In spite of the notion that there may be other unrecognised metabolic or environmental risk factors, secular changes in mortality from coronary disease which are occurring worldwide, and logistic function studies based on primary and secondary follow-up studies of coronary patients suggest that relatively small changes in the incidence of hyperlipidaemia and hypertension, and in smoking habits, may have considerable effects on coronary morbidity and mortality. It is likely that the coronary epidemic can be controlled without necessarily identifying and controlling all possible risk factors.

Family history

Physicians often encounter patients or healthy people who are apprehensive about a family history of coronary disease. Coronary patients may attribute

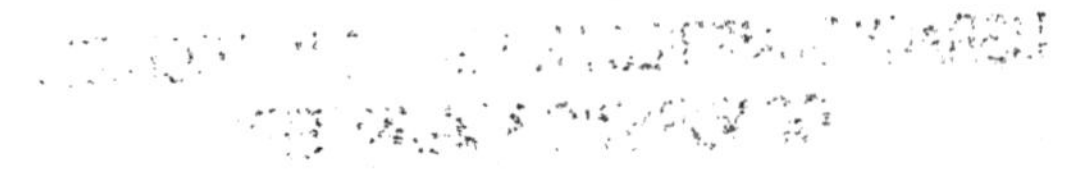

their illness to a family propensity, while the healthy person, reporting a recent coronary event in the family, may be apprehensive about his or her future health. We are faced with a challenge in helping these patients, a challenge which must be met realistically and as fairly as possible.

A review of the literature finds conflicting evidence that there is a primary genetic factor at the basis of coronary proneness. The various studies reported have been equivocal and opinions have been divided (Jorde & Williams 1988). In our own case-history study of risk factors in patients under 60 years with a first myocardial infarction, we found hypertension, hyperlipidaemia and cigarette smoking to be disproportionately and independently present (Mulcahy et al 1967, Mulcahy et al 1969), but we did not find a positive family history, in the absence of other risk factors, to be an independent factor. This is not to say that coronary heart disease does not aggregate in some families. Indeed it does, but this is not surprising when one considers the high prevalence of coronary heart disease in the community, and when one considers the common sharing of eating, smoking and exercise habits among parents and siblings, and the family tendency to hypertension and diabetes. It is, of course, likely that some families are more vulnerable to the adverse effects of smoking, lack of exercise and a high fat diet. As such, a susceptibility to coronary disease may be a polygenic one, depending on exposure and response to known and unknown risk factors rather than an independent monogenic trait. However, about one in 500 families are genetically deficient or lacking in LDL receptors, either in the relatively common heterozygous form or the rare homozygous form.

A positive family history for heart disease does deserve our attention, but mainly because of the need to seek out and eliminate coronary risk factors. With such an approach, both in primary and secondary prevention, it seems reasonable to adopt an optimistic line of reassurance about a positive family history.

REFERENCES

Ball K P, Hanington E, McAllen P M et al 1965 Low-fat diet in myocardial infarction. Lancet 2:501-504

Bierenbaum M L, Fleischman A I, Green D P et al 1970 The five year experience of modified fat diets on younger men with coronary heart disease. Circulation 42:943-952

Buring J E, Evans D A, Fiofe M, Rosner B, Hennekens C H 1987 Occupations and risk of death from coronary heart disease. Journal of the American Medical Association 258:791-792

Canner P L, Berge K G, Wnger N K et al 1986 Fifteen year mortality in Coronary Drug Project patients: long-term benefit with niacin. Journal of the American College of Cardiology 8:1245-1255

Connolly D C, Eleveback L R, Oxman H A 1983 Coronary heart disease in residents of Rochester, Minnesota, 1950-1975 111. Effect of hypertension and its treatment on survival of patients with coronary artery disease. Mayo Clinic Proceedings 58:259-264

Daly L E, Graham I M, Hickey N, Mulcahy R 1985 Does stopping smoking delay onset of angina after infarction? British Medical Journal 291:935-937

Graham I M, Mulcahy R, Hickey N, Daly L 1978 Effect of hypertension and its treatment on progress after myocardial infarction. In: Hjalmarson H, Wilhelmsen L (eds) Acute and Long-term Medical Management of Myocardial Infarction. Lindgren Molndal, pp 279-284

Hamalainen H, Luurila O J, Kallio V, Knuts L-R, Arstila M, Hakkila J 1989 Long-term reduction in sudden deaths after a multifactorial intervention programme in patients with myocardial infarction: ten year results of a controlled investigation. European Heart Journal 10:55-62

Hansen P F, Geill T, Lund E 1962 Dietary fats and thrombosis. Lancet 2:1193-1194

Jorde L B, Williams R R 1988 Relation between family history of coronary artery disease and coronary risk variables. American Journal of Cardiology 62:708-713

Kallio V, Hamalainen H, Hokkila J, Luurila O J 1979 Reduction in sudden deaths by a multifactorial intervention programme after acute myocardial infarction. Lancet 2: 1091-1094

Kannel W B, McGee D I, Castelli W P 1984 Latest perspectives on cigarette smoking and cardiovascular disease: The Framingham Study. Journal of Cardiac Rehabilitation 4:267-277

Keys A, Aravanis C, Blackburn H et al 1966 Epidemiological studies related to coronary heart disease: characteristics of men aged 40-59 in seven countries. Tampere

Leren P 1970 The Oslo diet-heart study. Eleven-year report. Circulation 42:935-942

Medical Research Council 1968 Controlled trial of soya-bean oil in myocardial infarction. Lancet 2:693-699

Morrison L M 1960 Diet in coronary atherosclerosis. Journal of the American Medical Association 173:884-888

Mulcahy R 1983 Influence of cigarette smoking on morbidity and mortality after myocardial infarction. British Heart Journal 49:410-415

Mulcahy R, Hickey N, Maurer B 1967 Coronary heart disease in women. Study of risk factors in 100 patients less than 60 years of age. Circulation 36:577-586

Mulcahy R, Hickey N, Maurer B 1969 Coronary heart disease. A study of risk factors in 400 patients under 60 years. Geriatrics 24:106-114

Mulcahy R, Daly L, Graham I, Hickey N 1984 Level of education, coronary risk factors and cardiovascular disease. Irish Medical Journal 77:316-318

Multiple Risk Factor Intervention Trial Research Group 1982 Multiple risk factor intervention trial: risk factor changes and mortality. Journal of the American Medical Association 248:1465-1477

Oldridge N B, Guyatt G H, Fischer M E, Rimm A A 1988 Cardiac rehabilitation after myocardial infarction. Combined experience of randomized clinical trials. Journal of the American Medical Association 260:945-950

Phillips A N, Shaper A G, Pocock S J, Walker M, MacFarlane P W 1988. The role of risk factors in heart attack occurring in men with pre-existing ischaemic heart disease. British Heart Journal 60:404-410

Rose G, Marmot M G 1981 Social class and coronary heart disease. British Heart Journal 45:13-19

Rose G A, Thomsom W B, Williams R T 1965 Corn oil in treatment of ischaemic heart disease. British Medical Journal 24:1159-1191

World Health Organization 1989. Coronary heart disease mortality for thirty six countries. World Health Organization, Geneva, (personal communication).

FURTHER READING

Borhani NO 1985 Prevention of coronary heart disease in practice. Implications of the results of recent clinical trials. Journal of the American Medical Association 254:257-262

European Atherosclerosis Society 1987 A strategy for the prevention of coronary heart disease. European Heart Journal 8:77-81

Mulcahy R 1987 The role of the general practitioner in the prevention of coronary heart disease. In: Sandler G. (ed) Coronary Heart Disease. MTP Press, Lancaster, 27-57

World Health Organization 1985 Primary prevention of coronary heart disease. Report on a World Health Organization meeting. Euro-reports and studies 98. Copenhagen.

World Health Organization 1982 Prevention of coronary heart disease. Technical Report Series 678, WHO, Geneva

4. Classification and clinical presentation of coronary heart disease

Coronary artery disease is a pathological term signifying atherosclerosis of one or more of the coronary arteries. Coronary heart disease is a clinical term indicating symptomatic coronary artery disease. In fact, a small proportion of patients, perhaps less than 5%, present with some or all of the clinical features of coronary heart disease, but may have little or nothing to show in the coronary arteries on angiography or at pathological examination (Castello et al 1990). In such cases we must postulate some unusual mechanism, such as arterial spasm or rapid resolution of a localised thrombus.

CLASSIFYING CORONARY HEART DISEASE

A simple classification of coronary artery and coronary heart disease is shown in Fig. 4.1 below.

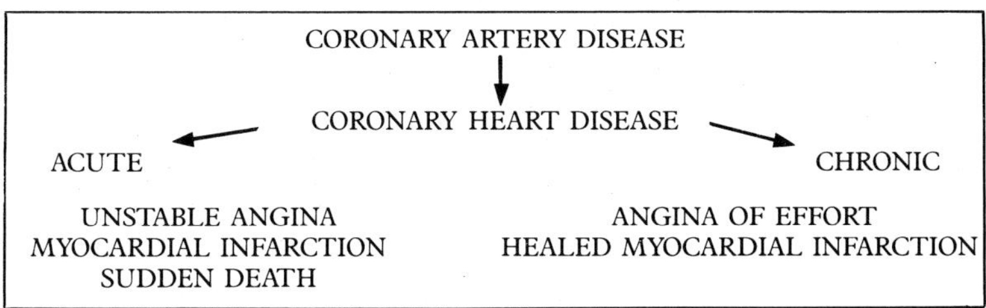

Fig. 4.1 Classifying coronary artery and coronary heart disease.

Unstable angina

This term is widely employed to include a number of different acute coronary syndromes which may presage a high risk of myocardial infarction or sudden death. Other terms previously or currently employed are angina decubitus, pre-infarction syndrome, intermediate coronary syndrome and acute coronary insufficiency. Because unstable angina indicates a high risk of early myocardial infarction or sudden death, its recognition is important to ensure that threatened patients are under conventional coronary care, at least until symptoms have subsided. It is our custom to subdivide unstable angina into the following categories:

1. Recent (less than one month) onset of angina of effort
2. Angina of effort of increasing severity (crescendo angina)
3. Recurring rest pain, with or without previous angina.

This latter presentation we call acute coronary insufficiency. This includes patients with variant or Prinzmetal angina.

Patients with unstable angina have by definition no evidence of recent heart muscle necrosis as confirmed by negative enzyme rise, and do not show the classical acute ECG changes of myocardial infarction. They may show recent or serial STT changes of ischaemia. These changes are labile and vary in character from acute T-wave inversion, STT depression, ST elevation and peaking of T-waves. In a minority of cases of acute coronary insufficiency, the STT elevation may be marked, very labile and associated with severe recurring rest pain. This fairly clearly defined syndrome is called Prinzmetal or variant angina. It is believed to presage a greater risk of infarction or sudden death. Patients with acute coronary insufficiency may present without ECG changes. In such cases, one is dependent on careful history taking, so that caution must be observed to ensure that the patients are kept under observation until the symptoms subside.

Unstable angina in one form or another frequently precedes acute infarction or sudden death. In the rehabilitation of patients with coronary heart disease, it is routine practice to alert patients and family members about the significance of worsening angina of effort or of cardiac pain at rest. Immediate referral to the family doctor or, preferably, to the emergency department of the nearest hospital, is advised under such circumstances.

Myocardial infarction

The classical diagnostic features are prolonged cardiac pain at rest, a more than two-fold increase in the cardiac enzymes—creatine kinase (CK), glutamic-oxalacetic transferase (GOT) and lactic dehydrogenase (LDH)—and STT elevation, with or without reciprocal changes of STT depression in the contralateral leads, followed subsequently by T-wave inversion and the appearance of pathological Q-waves. The picture varies widely with great variations in the severity, duration and location of pain, and with enzyme changes which depend largely on the extent of the infarction and on the duration of time since the onset of the attack. ECG changes are also variable, with delay in onset of STT changes or rarely, without any ECG changes, with no evidence of subsequent Q-waves and, in some patients, with a rapid return of the ECG changes to normal. The latter outcome is generally associated with early revascularisation and may be more frequently found after thrombolytic therapy.

The extent of infarction varies considerably and largely determines the immediate and the subsequent prognosis in terms of complications and death. The presence of previous infarction adds to the prognostic significance of a fresh attack, because of the extent of left ventricular impairment. Hence the importance of paying special attention to the pre-ention of further episodes of infarction as part of the rehabilitation process.

Supraventricular and life threatening ventricular arrhythmias, manifestations of heart block, including atrioventricular dissociation and bundle branch block, cardiogenic shock, and acute left ventricular failure are complications of acute myocardial infarction which require anticipation and treatment in the coronary care unit. These complications are rare as maniestations of unstable angina, unless the patient has suffered significant heart muscle damage in the past. Other less common complications include ventricular rupture, mitral regurgitation, and pulmonary and systemic embolisation. Pericarditis is a frequent but not a serious complication. It may be troublesome when it tends to recur. It is then described as Dressler's syndrome.

Patients are subject to psychological complications when admitted with unstable angina or myocardial infarction. Initially, anxiety is common. Less commonly, at the early stages, depression and denial may occur.

Sudden death

Sudden death is, for the purpose of this monograph, defined as instantaneous and unexpected death of non-traumatic origin. However, in epidemiological parlance, sudden death is generally described as unexpected death occurring within 24 hours. The forensic pathologists will confirm that sudden unexpected death of non-traumatic origin in the community can be attributed to heart disease in 80-90% of cases (Lown 1984). While sudden cardiac death may occur with valvular disease, cardiomyopathies, congenital lesions of the coronary vessels and of other cardiac structures, in the majority of cases extensive disease of the coronary vessels will be evident. The mechanism of sudden death in patients with coronary heart disease can be attributed to ventricular fibrillation in 90% of cases, although heart block and asystole may be the mechanism, particularly in patients with extensive heart muscle damage.

For purposes of rehabilitation it is important to identify predictors of sudden death in patients with angina or in survivors of myocardial infarction. These include extensive left ventricular impairment and the presence of certain ventricular arrhythmias, including frequent, pairs or salvoes of ventricular ectopic beats, and multifocal ectopics. Bouts of ventricular tachycardia, particularly when symptomatic or when associated with severe left ventricular impairment, have a sinister significance. Sudden death is a common cause of death among patients who recover from a myocardial infarction. In our follow-up study we found that 40% of deaths are sudden and unexpected during the first year after an infarction but the proportion of sudden deaths to deaths from fresh myocardial infarction, and other vascular and non-vascular causes, falls to 20% or less after ten to 15 years (Daly et al 1987).

The prospect of a sudden demise is a common cause of anxiety among patients after a heart attack. Such anxiety often resolves with adequate reassurance and explanation, particularly if the patient perceives that measures are being taken to avoid recurrence of further coronary episodes.

Angina of effort

By definition, angina of effort is a chronic form of coronary heart disease in that the pain on effort is constant in relation to myocardial oxygen demands. Angina may improve or resolve, particularly in response to coronary surgery and anti-anginal drugs. Angina may change in intensity over the years, and may resolve spontaneously in patients who are treated conservatively by risk factor modification and graduated exercise programmes (Redwood et al 1972, Kennedy et al 1976). Many patients will, however, complain of angina of effort of constant intensity over many months or years. In others it may fluctuate in intensity, within certain limits, depending on climatic, behavioural and psychological factors, and on medication.

Patients with chronic angina of effort are at higher risk of myocardial infarction and sudden death than apparently healthy people, but nevertheless the prognosis can be quite good over the long term if they have good left ventricular function, if they are free of obvious coronary risk factors, if they maintain a satisfactory aerobic exercise programme, and if they have no critical atherosclerotic plaques in the left main stem or the proximal left anterior descending vessel. Angina becomes prognostically more sinister, and may presage early myocardial infarction or sudden death, when it becomes more frequent, more prolonged and more severe in response to effort, or when it is of recent onset. As such, it is included among the pre-infarction or unstable angina syndromes.

Silent ischaemia

Silent ischaemia has been receiving increasing attention recently (Fox 1988, Singh 1988, Mulcahy et al 1989, Kannel 1989) and may pose a problem in management during the rehabilitation and follow-up phase. It is almost invariably manifested by episodes of STT depression being detected during exercise testing and Holter monitoring. By definition, transient ischaemic changes occur without accompanying anginal pain or chest discomfort. Silent ischaemia is almost invariably found in the presence of significant coronary artery disease and probably does not differ in prognostic significance from symptomatic ischaemia. ST elevation is extremely rare, except in those with unstable angina or with previous myocardial infarction.

Conventional treatment with anti-anginal drugs, particularly beta-blockers, will reduce the frequency, duration and magnitude of the STT changes. Whether such drugs improve prognosis is a moot point. While the natural history of silent and symptomatic ischaemia appears to be similar in prognostic terms, controversy remains about the significance of the silent episodes and about their optimum management. Nor is there any reliable information about the beneficial effects, if any, of exercise programmes and risk factor modification on the frequency of the silent episodes.

Until a clearer picture emerges of the diagnostic and prognostic significance of silent ischaemia, and until therapeutic indications have been clarified, it is probably best to advise a conservative approach to management as long as associated symptomatic episodes are not disabling and as long as routine risk factor modification and exercise training are prescribed. Surgery or angioplasty may be considered in the presence of marked ECG changes and of associated disabling angina of effort, and where the coronary morphology is deemed suitable at coronary angiography.

Healed myocardial infarction

The prognosis of patients with longstanding scarring of the myocardium depends on the extent of heart damage and the risks of recurring infarction. Most patients have a history of previous myocardial infarction but about 20% of subjects observed during community screening programmes to have an old myocardial infarction in the ECG will be unaware of such an episode (Margolis et al 1973). These patients with silent infarctions can be included in the same prognostic category as those with a previous history, the prognosis largely depending on the extent of heart muscle damage.

DIAGNOSIS OF CORONARY HEART DISEASE

The gold standard of diagnosis remains a history of pain. While the nature of the pain may vary considerably in severity, location, duration, radiation and character, and in its mode of onset, the pain of angina or myocardial infarction generally exhibits a sufficient number of characteristic features to attract, at the least, a strong suspicion of its presence. However, accurate interpretation requires diligence and experience on the part of the physician, but the experienced and conscientious physician will seldom err, even in the presence of a normal or near normal ECG, or with normal enzymes and other clinical and investigative findings. There is a latter day view that the gold standard of diagnosis is based on angiographic findings. However, the angiogram merely confirms the extent, severity and location of the atherosclerotic process. It does not inform us of the presence of clinically manifest disease. Anyhow, its findings are seldom available at the most crucial moments of diagnosis, when the patient is seen in the community or in the emergency department of a hospital.

It is important that patients and family members should be aware of the nature of cardiac pain and that they can readily differentiate cardiac pain from the many non-specific heart pains, including left submammary pain, which are so frequent after myocardial infarction and heart surgery, and which are commonly the cause of anxiety and depression in poorly informed patients. The presence of typical cardiac pain occurring under exceptional circumstances of exercise or at rest should be reported immediately to the patient's physician. Cardiac enzymes will assist in identifying the presence and extent of recent heart necrosis, while the resting ECG will confirm the presence of active ischaemia or of old or recent myocardial infarction. The resting ECG does lack sensitivity, particularly in the case of angina of effort, where there is little or no heart muscle damage. In a minority of cases the exercise ECG may show equivocal or negative results in patients with chronic angina, or may be unhelpful because of confounding factors. In such an event, we may require to perform a thallium exercise test to identify the site, extent and duration of the ischaemic lesion. A thallium exercise ECG may also be indicated before heart surgery and angioplasty to confirm the site of ischaemia.

The resting ECG may also lack sensitivity in patients with unstable angina or myocardial infarction, particularly in the early stages. A resting thallium test may be helpful in such patients to identify the site and location of the lesion, and a pyrophosphate scan of the myocardium, if performed within four to seven days of its onset, may identify a fresh infarction.

A symptom-limited or maximum exercise ECG is not infrequently advised in patients with unstable angina, particularly after symptoms have subsided. A positive test may be helpful in establishing the diagnosis but a negative test must not be deemed to rule out coronary disease. Patients with unstable angina, and particularly the patients with recurring rest pain, without a history of chronic angina of effort, frequently have a normal exercise ECG, due to the poor sensitivity of stress tests in this coronary syndrome.

PROGNOSIS

In reaching a prognosis in relation to rehabilitation and longterm management, the single most important index remains the degree of left ventricular impairment. Assessment of left ventricular function from the management and prognostic points of view is essentially a clinical matter. It can be measured in terms of history of left ventricular failure, heart size clinically and on X-ray, the presence of a third heart sound, and a poor exercise capacity during normal activities and as measured on the treadmill. Left ventricular function can also be quantified by measuring the left ventricular dimensions and ejection fraction, and the resting and exercise left ventricular end diastolic pressure, by means of echocardiography, MUGA scan, and left heart catheterisation and ventriculography. These tests will help to quantify the degree of left ventricular impairment and are useful in longterm management, and in measuring prognosis and response to treatment. Nevertheless, from the practical management point of view, they are not essential in most patients who are subjected to a careful clinical assessment of left ventricular function.

INVESTIGATIONS

The following investigations are available in assisting the clinician to arrive at a diagnosis of coronary heart disease, to establish prognosis and risk stratification, and to measure response to treatment:

cardiac enzymes
ECG
exercise stress test
resting and exercise thallium 201
dipyridamole stress test and atrial pacing
chest X-ray
echocardiogram
MUGA scan
left and right catheter studies
ventriculography
computer assisted tomography
magnetic resonance imaging

CARDIAC INVESTIGATIONS—THEIR INDICATIONS, LIMITATIONS AND POSSIBLE ADVERSE EFFECTS

Cardiac enzymes

These enzymes include creatine kinase (CK), glutamic—oxalacetic transferase (GOT) and lactic dehydrogenase (LDH). GOT and LDH are not specific for myocardial muscle because of their presence in many other organs, and in blood and skeletal muscles. CK is more specific but nevertheless CK can rise in other unrelated conditions. Enzymes which are specific to heart muscle damage are the LDH1 fraction and the CK—MB isoenzyme fraction.

The enzyme rise following myocardial infarction may be delayed according to the enzyme under study. CK appears within 4 to 8 hours, GOT within 8 to 12 hours and LDH within 24 to 48 hours. Peak values also vary, with CK peaking at 12 to 24 hours, GOT at 18 to 36 hours, and LDH at 3 to 6 days. Peak values will give useful information about infarct size and will assist in subsequent risk stratification, but caution is required to outrule confounding non-cardiac sources which may add to the enzyme rise.

The electrocardiogram

The 12-lead electrocardiogram is a standard diagnostic method to detect cardiac arrhythmias and conduction disorders. It is particularly valuable in the diagnosis of myocardial ischaemia and infarction. It contributes to the diagnosis of pericarditis, ventricular and atrial hypertrophy, and the effects of certain drugs, disturbances of electrolyte balance, and of some systemic diseases of the heart.

It is useful in checking pacemaker function and may provide information about the extent of heart muscle damage and hence about the immediate and longterm prognosis. However, its sensitivity is not 100% and it is frequently negative in patients with chronic angina, where there is normal or near normal heart muscle. It may show no abnormalities in patients with recent or previous unstable angina or myocardial infarction.

Holter monitor

Here the ECG is recorded continuously, generally over a 24 hour period. The recordings are stored in a cassette attached to the patient. They are subsequently analysed by a computer and recorded on a printout. A Holter recording is useful to detect the frequency and nature of arrhythmias and to detect ischaemic episodes, whether silent or symptomatic.

Exercise stress test

There are a number of instruments employed in stress testing, but the commonest method nowadays is the treadmill, although the bicycle ergometer is still widely used. A number of well known protocols have been established and are used in performing the test. The 12 standard leads are now customary but other special leads are occasionally used, especially for research purposes. The exercise test is performed to measure the subject's exercise capacity, to measure the heart rate and blood pressure response to exercise, and to detect exercise-induced ECG changes of ischaemia, arrhythmias and conduction defects. Exercise testing is useful in diagnosis, prognosis and in controlling treatment. It is particularly valuable in establishing the presence of exercise-induced ischaemia and is largely used nowadays in the diagnosis of chest pain, in the assessment of the extent and severity of ischaemia, and in deciding on the need for coronary angiography. It is used in planning a rehabilitation and training programme, and in monitoring the progress of training. The effect of exercise on heart rate, ECG changes, and blood pressure provides important information about risk stratification based on left ventricular function, and a tendency to arrhythmias and conduction defects. It is commonly employed after recovery from myocardial infarction for these purposes. The sensitivity and specificity of the exercise test in high risk populations, such as patients attending hospital, is satisfactory but it is unsatisfactory in apparently healthy populations. It is therefore unsuitable for routine screening purposes. In interpreting an exercise test, precautions must be taken to ensure that apparent abnormalities are not artefactual or due to causes other than coronary heart disease. There are contradictions to the exercise test, particularly active unstable angina with persisting rest pain, congestive heart failure, severe aortic stenosis, heart block and life-threatening arrhythmias.

Exercise thallium 201 test

In certain patients, the routine exercise stress test may be unsatisfactory for a number of reasons, including the presence of abnormalities in the resting tracings. In this case an exercise thallium 201 test may be indicated. The detection of thallium 201, the distribution of which in the heart is dependent upon regional perfusion, requires scintigraphy using a scintillation camera. When thallium is injected during exercise, a perfusion defect is identified by a reduced concentration in the myocardium. If the perfusion defect is caused by transient ischaemia, repeated imaging will show a return to normal perfusion after a few hours. No change will be noted if the perfusion defect is due to a healed infarct or to other permanent myocardial damage. The location of the ischaemia may give a clue to the artery or arteries involved, although coronary arteriography is needed to provide more specific and reliable information about this. Thallium scintigraphy is proving useful in identifying the 'culprit lesion' in those with angina and multi-vessel disease. This allows for the correct choice of lesion to be angioplastied, now that angioplasty is being performed in those with more complex disease. The thallium 201 exercise test is a useful adjunct to conventional exercise testing but requires more time and needs expensive equipment.

Dipyridamole stress test and atrial pacing

In patients who are unable to exercise for one reason or another, a standard intravenous dose of dipyridamole will lead to transient tachycardia and thus will simulate a submaximal exercise test. Its sensitivity and specificity are unreliable and, as an alternative to more conventional stress testing, it is not generally recommended. An increase in heart rate can be induced by atrial pacing, which is also occasionally used instead of the more conventional stress test.

The chest X-ray

The chest X-ray may provide useful information in assessing prognosis. There is a close correlation between heart size as measured radiologically and prognosis in patients with chronic coronary disease and other cardiac conditions. Structural changes in the heart and intrathoracic vessels may also be apparent from the X-ray and may assist in diagnosis. Apart from the conventional postero-anterior film, lateral views may be required, and will help in the diagnosis of chamber hypertrophy. Lateral views also help to confirm that apparent cardiomegaly in the postero-anterior film is not caused by a thoracic cage anomaly or some other non-cardiac cause. The chest X-ray is useful in patients with various types of heart disease in identifying pulmonary venous congestion and pulmonary oedema. Localised pulmonary oligaemia may suggest pulmonary embolism.

Fluoroscopy, previously widely employed to identify selective chamber enlargement and other abnormalities of cardiac and vascular silhouettes, is now less frequently used. It is useful in identifying calcification of the cardiac structures, including the pericardium, and, using an image intensifier, is necessary for the insertion of pacing wires and other cardiac catheters. Deeply penetrating chest films and image intensification are particularly useful in identifying calcification. Routine fluoroscopy is now rarely employed.

Echocardiography

Echocardiography is perhaps the most useful non-invasive investigation introduced in cardiology during the past 20 years. This ultrasound technique can measure certain structural and functional cardiac phenomena through images obtained from sound frequencies reflected from the cardiac structures. There are two methods employed, M-mode and two-dimensional echocardiography.

The M-mode echocardiogram provides information about the dimensions of the heart cavities and walls, about valve structure and function, and about the pericardial space and other intracardiac structures. The usefulness of the technique is somewhat limited in some instances, because of inaccessibility of parts of the heart to the probe.

Two-dimensional echocardiography, as well as identifying the cardiac structures, also measures global and regional ventricular function, ejection fraction, ventricular wall thickness, and a variety of intracavitary masses, congenital malformations, pericardial disease and aneurysm. With the addition of a Doppler signal, blood flow can be measured and information can be provided about shunts, valve stenosis and incompetence, and about cardiac output. A coloured Doppler is particularly useful to measure patterns of blood flow and pressure gradients across valves.

Echocardiography is currently not adequate to identify disease in the coronary arteries, and is frequently unsatisfactory in patients with chronic lung disease because of the presence of air between the transducer and the heart. Echocardiography is replacing other more complex invasive investigations, particularly in children.

Multiple gated acquisition scan (MUGA)

With this technique, using a gamma camera, the cardiac chambers can be visualised and ventricular function can be assessed visually and quantitatively by tagging the red blood cells with technetium-99m. After several minutes, when there is complete mixing of the technetium, several heart beats are combined to depict a typical cycle during the imaging period. This gives information, not only about left and right ventricular function but also about segmental wall motion. It can identify areas of diminished or absent function in the left ventricle. MUGA scanning is mainly of value in quantifying cardiac function at rest and after exercise, and is therefore useful in measuring left ventricular function and in assessing the effects of treatment.

Pyrophosphate scan

This technique is not often used but may be required to identify recent myocardial infarction, if the clinical, ECG, and enzyme data are equivocal. Unfortunately the technique has poor specificity and sensitivity. It seldom adds useful information to clinical judgement and more conventional investigations.

Cardiac catheterisation and ventriculography

Cardiac catheterisation is widely used in the diagnosis of heart disease, and in identifying and quantifying haemodynamic abnormalities. The procedure is carried out under image intensification. It is useful in investigating the right side of the heart and the pulmonary circulation through the venous system, or the left side of the heart and the aortic structures through the femoral or antecubital artery. This technique can be used to measure pressures in the vessels and cardiac chambers, to measure cardiac output and to introduce opaque material into the cardiac chambers (ventriculography) and into the coronary arteries and other vessels (angiography). Coronary angiography identifies the extent, severity and location of coronary artery disease, although the severity of individual lesions cannot be estimated with absolute precision. Coronary angiography is absolutely essential to identify the location and severity of critical obstructive lesions in the coronary vessels before undertaking angioplasty or coronary artery surgery.

Ventriculography, or the introduction of dye into the left ventricle, gives useful information about left ventricular function and about localised abnormalities of left ventricular muscle, including aneurysm formation. As such, it may overlap the information provided by echocardiography and by MUGA scanning.

Computer assisted tomography

In general, computer assisted tomography scanning is of very limited value in the diagnosis and management of heart disease, apart from the diagnosis of dissecting aneurysm of the aorta. It may be useful in the diagnosis of unusual structures, such as pericardial tumours or unusual intracavity or heart muscle masses. Echocardiography is more effective and more easily available to identify such unusual anomalies.

Magnetic resonance imaging

Nuclear magnetic resonance imaging techniques rely on a powerful magnetic field and on radiowaves to form an image of a slice in a chosen plane through the patient. The images are of very high resolution and can be used to demonstrate clearly the anatomy, function, and blood flow of the heart. Its use allows invasive investigation to be avoided in some instances, and can provide important supplemental information in patients with various forms of heart disease. It is possible to image coronary artery by-pass grafts and to determine their patency, and it is likely that in the future it may be useful in studying blood flow in coronary arteries and grafts.

REFERENCES

Castello R, Alegria E, Merino A, Fidalgo M L, Martinez-Caro D 1990 The value of exercise testing in patients with coronary artery spasm. American Heart Journal 119:259-263

Daly L, Hickey N, Graham I M, Mulcahy R 1987 Predictors of sudden death up to 18 years after a first attack of unstable angina or myocardial infarction. British Heart Journal 58:567-571

Fox K M 1988 Silent ischaemia: clinical implications in 1988. British Heart Journal 60:363-366

Kannel W B 1989 Detection and management of patients with silent myocardial ischaemia. American Heart Journal 117:221-226

Kennedy C C, Spiekerman R E, Lindsay M I Jr et al 1976 One-year graduated exercise program for men with angina pectoris. Evaluation by physiologic studies and coronary arteriography. Mayo Clinic Proceedings 51:231-236

Lown B 1984 Cardiovascular collapse and sudden cardiac death. In: Braunwald E (ed) Heart disease: a textbook of cardiovascular medicine, 2nd ed. Saunders, Philadelphia pp 774-806

Margolis J R, Kannel W B, Feinleib M, Dawber T R, McNamara P M 1973 Clinical features of unrecognised myocardial infarction—silent and symptomatic. The Framingham Study. American Journal of Cardiology 32:1-7

Mulcahy D, Keegan J, Sparrow J, Park A, Wright C, Fox K 1989 Ischaemia in the ambulatory setting—the total ischaemic burden: relation to exercise testing and investigative and therapeutic implications. Journal of the American College of Cardiology 14:1166-1172

Redwood D R, Rosing D R, Epstein S E 1972 Circulatory and symptomatic effects of physical training in patients with coronary-artery disease and angina pectoris. New England Journal of Medicine 286:959-965

Singh (ed) 1988 Silent myocardial ischaemia and angina: prevalence, diagnostic and therapeutic significance. Pergamon Press, Oxford

FURTHER READING

World Health Organization 1988 Appropriate diagnostic technology in the management of cardiovascular diseases. Report of an Expert Committee, Technical Report Series 772, WHO, Geneva

SECTION 2

Principles of rehabilitation

5. Principles of rehabilitation

The medical and psychological impact of coronary heart disease and the chronic, often progressive nature of atherosclerosis, create circumstances which require a special and exceptional rehabilitation approach. This approach differs fundamentally from the rehabilitation approach to most other acute and chronic illnesses. Coronary heart disease frequently presents suddenly and without warning, and is usually a cause of significant anxiety, loss of security and self esteem, and an abrupt reminder of one's mortality. Its impact is aggravated by the victim's ignorance of a perceived or obvious cause, and by the knowledge that there is a propensity to further events and particularly to sudden unforeseen death. Anxiety and depression are further aggravated by the public perception of the poor outlook in terms of recovery and return to normal life which was so evident in the past and which still prevails, despite the dramatic changes in management, and the shedding of negative and restrictive professional attitudes in recent years.

Bearing in mind these aspects of the nature and significance of coronary heart disease, a successful rehabilitation philosophy must be adopted with the following objectives in view:

1. A return to a normal social, recreational, sexual and professional life
2. Maintaining or improving the subject's quality of life
3. Ensuring complete psychological recovery
4. Reducing subsequent morbidity and mortality, with particular emphasis on reducing the risk of sudden death or of further coronary events through risk factor intervention, exercise programmes, surgery and appropriate medication
5. Ensuring that the benefits of rehabilitation are sustained over time, to encourage longterm compliance, desirable life-style changes and to obviate recidivism
6. Ensuring that no harm is effected by the rehabilitation process
7. Providing cost effective programmes.

COST EFFICACY

The cost efficacy of coronary rehabilitation is crucial if programmes are to be widely adopted and if their benefits are to be enjoyed by the large number of patients surviving myocardial infarction or heart surgery, or who are suffering from chronic angina of effort. It is estimated that 550,000 die from coronary heart disease in the United States every year (Consensus Conference 1985), while more than 1,000,000 will survive a heart attack. Only some of these patients receive the benefits of rehabilitation measures. Few enjoy programmes satisfying all the above objectives. Worldwide rehabilitation facilities are at best patchy and poorly co-ordinated and, as a general rule, it is likely that effective rehabilitation services are either inadequate or totally lacking in western countries (Worcester 1986). If one is to judge by the interest shown by contemporary cardiologists in this aspect of heart disease, one would be forgiven for thinking that their commitment was more in the breach than in the observance.

It is evident from our experience of cardiac rehabilitation over the last 24 years, and from the experience of other workers, that cost-effective rehabilitation services can be provided without the need for special facilities in terms of staff, equipment and space, and without the expenditure of extra funds over and above those required to maintain the usual services of a district or teaching hospital. Current rehabilitation programmes vary in complexity and cost, from the simplest type of clinically orientated outpatient facility with group or home-based exercise programmes, to specially equipped institutions providing a wealth of diagnostic and therapeutic facilities. A minority of patients may require special rehabilitation procedures, particularly in relation to psychological adjustment, exercise compliance, and management of complications, but the great majority of myocardial infarction and surgical survivors can be as effectively managed by an informal rehabilitation programme guided by a group of health professionals derived from the normal cardiological team in the hospital. Cost-effective rehabilitation should be part of the routine cardiological practice in all our hospitals, and its perception as a specialised discipline requiring special facilities, training and staff, is simply retarding the adoption of the proper longterm care of our patients with coronary heart disease.

REHABILITATION OBJECTIVES

How do we measure successful outcome of rehabilitation programmes in patients with coronary heart disease? In early years, we were mostly concerned with the end-points of return to work and adopting exercise programmes. The objectives have widened in scope in recent years to include attempts to reduce delayed symptoms and complications, and to reduce the risk of further fatal and non-fatal coronary episodes through risk factor intervention, exercise programmes, surgery and medication. There is increasing emphasis on the need to improve quality of life through appropriate psychosocial adjustments and life-style changes. Social support and family involvement will enhance good psychosocial adjustment and will contribute to good health promotional education and practices within the family and the community. An active rehabilitation service will be instrumental in underlining the fact that good health promotional practices do not depend exclusively on advocacy by health professionals but require the full commitment, co-operation and understanding of the community as a whole.

Some rehabilitation objectives may be difficult to measure, such as quality of life and psychosocial adjustment. A routine interview with the patient will often tell us whether quality of life has improved following myocardial infarction. This is frequently the case when we employ effective rehabilitation procedures. A great variety of questionnaires have been employed to test quality of life but these questionnaires have their limitations and there is little agreement among physicians and psychologists about the best instruments to use. We now have a bewildering variety of questionnaires which have been advocated but, from the practical point of view, we need to employ such questionnaires only for research purposes.

Table 5.1 is a simple questionnaire which has been used by us and gives useful information about depression, anxiety, motivation and self-esteem.

Table 5.1 St Vincent's Hospital Quality of Life Questionnaire

We would like you to answer the following questions. Your answers will be treated in the strictest confidence and will only be seen by your physician and the cardiac staff.

Compared with before your heart illness, how do you rate yourself now as regards the following . . . (tick one box only).

	Much worse	Worse	No change	Better	Much better
1. Sleep	[ ]	[ ]	[ ]	[ ]	[ ]
2. Energy	[ ]	[ ]	[ ]	[ ]	[ ]
3. Worry or tension	[ ]	[ ]	[ ]	[ ]	[ ]
4. Happiness/contentment	[ ]	[ ]	[ ]	[ ]	[ ]
5. Confidence	[ ]	[ ]	[ ]	[ ]	[ ]
6. Sexual interest	[ ]	[ ]	[ ]	[ ]	[ ]
7. Sadness/depression	[ ]	[ ]	[ ]	[ ]	[ ]
8. General physical health	[ ]	[ ]	[ ]	[ ]	[ ]

RETURN TO WORK

Other objectives of rehabilitation may be jeopardised because of failure of compliance over time. One measure of success of compliance among younger patients is return to work after myocardial infarction or coronary artery surgery. This end-point has been extensively studied, and it is an indication of the success of modern cardiac rehabilitation that return to work rates, which were unusually low 30 years ago, have been reported to be as high as 90%, in some cases by the early 1970s (Mulcahy & Hickey 1970, Mulcahy et al 1988).

The reasons for delay or failure to return to work have been extensively studied and, in contrast to previous fears, have been attributed more frequently to social, psychological and personal factors rather than to disability from coronary disease or other organic conditions (Mulcahy 1976, Cay & Walker 1988). It is now well established that no occupation is contra-indicated on medical grounds in patients fully recovered from a myocardial infarction, and that careful risk factor modification will ensure that all patients, who are not seriously or permanently disabled, can be returned to their former occupations. Personnel in certain occupations who care for the safety of large numbers of people, such as bus and train drivers, and airline pilots, are currently barred from returning to work as a matter of public policy, but even in these occupations, with improving risk assessment, guidelines may prove to be more liberal in the future (Robinson & Mulcahy 1986).

REHABILITATION AMONG THE ELDERLY

Appropriate rehabilitation services should be available for coronary patients of all groups, including the elderly. The approach to rehabilitation may differ in detail, particularly in relation to return to work, but the principles of rehabilitation must remain the same, that is, a return to a normal good quality of life appropriate to the subject's circumstances and age. This must include risk factor modification, attention to non-cardiac causes of disability and adopting active aerobic exercise. It is as important for the 75-year-old man or woman who has recovered from a myocardial infarction to adopt active and regular aerobic exercise as it is for the young survivor of 40 years. In the case of the elderly, draconian measures aimed at risk factor modification should not be necessary and special care will be required in prescribing medication such as beta-blockers, diuretics and psychotropic drugs.

SELF-HELP GROUPS

Longterm compliance may be enhanced by the use of patient self-help groups. These groups or 'coronary clubs' are becoming more popular, and are already fully and widely established in a few countries (Konig 1978, Wenger 1981). Like other self-help groups, patients with coronary heart disease meet regularly to provide mutual support and encouragement. A doctor or other health professional may be in attendance and a continued education programme on all aspects of rehabilitation and longterm management may be provided. It is likely that such self-help groups are the most effective means of ensuring satisfactory compliance with desirable behaviourial change and risk factor modification.

REFERENCES

Cay E L, Walker D D 1988 Psychological factors and return to work. European Heart Journal 9:L74-81

Concensus Conference 1985. Lowering blood cholesterol to prevent heart disease. Journal of the American Medical Association 253:2080-2086

Konig K 1978 Organisation of rehabilitation centres. Advances in Cardiology 24:136-145

Mulcahy R 1976 The rehabilitation of patients with coronary heart disease. A clinician's view. In: Stocksmeier U (ed) Psychological approach to the rehabilitation of coronary patients. Springer-Verlag, Berlin pp 52-61

Mulcahy R, Hickey N 1970 The rehabilitation of patients with coronary heart disease. Scandinavian Journal of Rehabilitation 2-3:108

Mulcahy R, Kennedy C, Conroy R 1988 The longterm work record of post-infarction patients subjected to an informal rehabilitation and secondary prevention programme. European Heart Journal 9:L84-88

Robinson K, Mulcahy R 1986 Return to employment of professional truck drivers following myocardial infarction. Irish Medical Journal 72:31-33

Wenger N 1981 Rehabilitation in 'Coronary Clubs'. In: Konig K (ed) Progress in echocardiography and radionuclide methods. Lifelong rehabilitation in phase III. Waldrick, Frieburg, pp 91-93

Worcester M 1986 Cardiac rehabilitation programme in Australian Hospitals. National Heart Foundation of Australia, Canberra

FURTHER READING

Konig K, Denolin H, Dorossiev D (eds) 2nd edition 1983 Myocardial Infarction. How to Prevent, How to Rehabilitate: Scientific Council on Rehabilitation of Cardiac Patients, International Society and Federation of Cardiology, Boehringer Mannheim

Maisano G, Gobbato F, Julian D G, Mulcahy R 1988 Workshop on occupational cardiology therapy. European Heart Journal 9:L1-131

Wenger N K (ed) 1986 The Education of the Patient With Cardiac Disease in the Twenty-First Century. Le Jacq Publishing, New York

6. Early in-hospital rehabilitation

While the principles of cardiac rehabilitation are applicable to all patients with coronary heart disease, including those with chronic angina of effort and with previous myocardial infarction, those who are admitted to coronary care, and patients recovering from heart surgery, require specific early attention to ensure successful rehabilitation and return to a normal life. This chapter deals, firstly, with the management of patients with unstable angina and myocardial infarction admitted to coronary care, with special emphasis on early rehabilitation measures. The rest of the chapter deals with risk factor stratification and assessment of prognosis during and after recovery. Specific problems relating to rehabilitation after coronary artery surgery, angioplasty, valve surgery and transplantation are dealt with in Chapter 16.

EARLY REHABILITATION AFTER MYOCARDIAL INFARCTION

Patients admitted to coronary care with documented unstable angina or myocardial infarction are subjected to routine measures to prevent or limit the size of the infarct, and to anticipate, prevent and treat complications. A detailed discussion of routine coronary care procedures aimed at these objectives is not relevant to the subject of rehabilitation but, despite our preoccupation with such interventions, the prospects of satisfactory rehabilitation and recovery can be enhanced from the earliest time of admission. To ensure a satisfactory approach to early rehabilitation it is essential that all members of the coronary care staff, including nurses, resident doctors, and other medical personnel, should be educated in the principles and procedures of cardiac rehabilitation. It is imperative that the lead should come from the cardiologist and the sister in charge of the unit. In my experience, the charge sister plays a crucial role, both through precept and example, in encouraging an active approach to rehabilitation at this early stage in the patient's illness.

THE KEY ROLE OF COUNSELLING

Patients admitted with an acute myocardial infarction are almost invariably acutely anxious and perceive themselves as facing an unexpected catastrophe in their lives. Alleviation of anxiety can be optimised by early and good communication by the coronary care staff, by realistic reassurance, and by careful explanation of the activities and procedures which are part of routine coronary care. Good communication is not only a matter of verbal interchange between patient and staff. It can be enhanced by ensuring that patients are not isolated in the coronary care unit and that they are in close contact with the nurses and doctors. For this reason, I have always favoured open plan coronary care, except for special cases. In coronary care units designed with single rooms we should ensure that patients are not too isolated by closed and soundproof doors, and by remoteness from the nurses' station and from the normal ward activities.

In early discussion, when the patient's symptoms have subsided, it should be implicit in our explanations that full return to a normal life and to health is the rule in patients surviving a myocardial infarction. It is also useful at this stage to emphasise that the cause or causes of the heart attack can usually be identified, and that risk factor modification will play an important part in reducing the risk of further events. Equally, the availability of other treatment modalities, such as coronary artery surgery, angioplasty and drugs, should be stressed. One can often predict that a patient's quality of life may improve after myocardial infarction, with appropriate risk factor modification and exercise programmes.

Early ambulation

Leg, arm and breathing exercises should be commenced within 24 hours of admission, if the patient's condition allows. These exercises can be initiated and supervised by the physiotherapist, and should be maintained and encouraged by the nursing and the medical staffs. Early ambulation and group exercises in the recovery ward are also indicated. An emphasis at this stage of the value of exercise helps to highlight the importance of aerobic exercise in recovery and as part of the rehabilitation process and the future life-style prescription. Bed exercises are also designed to prevent thrombo-embolism and other adverse effects of immobilisation.

Risk factor modification

The later stages of hospitalisation provides an opportunity to identify risk factors and of advising about their control. It provides an opportunity for the social worker, dietitian and the physiotherapist, as well as the nursing and medical staff, to meet with the spouse and family members to discuss the patient's social, personal and professional background, and to advise about further management. It is mandatory that any life style or behaviourial changes prescribed for the patient, such as smoking cessation, blood pressure control or dietary modification, should be fully understood and should receive the full support, co-operation and, where indicated, the participation of the spouse and the family.

Early discharge

Early discharge after myocardial infarction is also helpful in speeding physical and psychological recovery. Patients with uncomplicated infarcts can usually be discharged home in less than seven days. Patients with extensive infarction complicated by arrhythmias, heart failure or other complications, may require a longer period in hospital, and may anticipate a slower recovery, but experience confirms that, in most complicated infarcts, the critical phase is passed within a few days, so prolonged hospitalisation is not often justified. Patients with unstable angina and persistent rest pain may also require a longer period of observation and treatment, but they are usually fit for discharge when the pain has resolved. There is little point in discharging patients to general medical wards or to special convalescent institutions at this stage. It is generally preferable to discharge patients to the security and familiarity of their home, if the home environment is satisfactory. It is also preferable to complete special investigations before discharge, if these can be done safely and appropriately at this stage. Returning patients to hospital for angiography and other special tests may retard rehabilitation by prolonging a sense of dependency and institutionalisation.

Early convalescence

Patients are advised to return to the rehabilitation and secondary prevention clinic within three weeks of discharge. This allows a reasonable period of early convalescence during which the patient is encouraged to adopt a graduated exercise programme and to return gradually to a normal social life. We have successfully encouraged patients at this stage to adopt a walking programme from the date of discharge, with the aim of walking about three miles (5 kilometres) daily by the time of the first outpatient visit. With clear instructions, and in all but the more complicated or disabled patients, this programme can be successfully achieved. Symptom-limited walking, graduated by intensity and distance, is prescribed during these early weeks. The symptomatic response to such exercise will give an accurate measure of the patient's exercise capacity, and will be reviewed at the first outpatient visit.

We have found home-planned exercise programmes based on walking to be the most satisfactory form of aerobic exercise during the early stages of convalescence, both in terms of compliance and safety. However, group exercises can be organised within the hospital setting or in special outpatient institutions. Ideally these group sessions should be combined with home exercise programmes. Group sessions do not require elaborate equipment or staffing, and they are useful in motivating patients to adopt more active lives. They may also introduce them to appropriate forms of exercise and acquaint them with the importance of risk factor modification.

In patients with the more severe degrees of left ventricular damage, exercise programmes should also be designed on a symptom-limited basis, but excessive caution is not justified and may have adverse psychological effects. Experience has shown that a satisfactory training effect can be achieved in such patients with an appropriate exercise programme (Squires et al 1987, Arvan 1988). Left ventricular function can improve significantly during the first two or three years in those who survive initial left ventricular damage, and the relatively bad prognosis associated with the more severe degrees of myocardial damage is mainly evident only during the first year or two after the initial event (Weinblatt et al 1968). A balanced programme of graduated exercise and regulated rest may eventually lead to a marked improvement in exercise capacity in such patients.

Before discharge from hospital, patient and family should be fully conversant with the need and the means of making desirable life-style changes to reduce the risk of delayed complications and the risk of subsequent recurring events. Apart from exercise, advice about smoking, control of hyperlipidaemia and obesity, adherence to prescribed medication for hypertension and diabetes should be clearly outlined, both verbally and by the use of appropriate literature. At this stage, the influence and intervention of the dietitian, the physiotherapist and social worker will reinforce the influence of the cardiologist. Psychologists are not infrequently employed to deal with psychological and mood problems, but, in our experience, most problems in this area are best dealt with by the cardiologist and by the rehabilitation team members, who can provide a broad-based approach encompassing clinical as well as psychological aspects of the patient's illness.

In advising patients and their families about necessary life-style changes to be adopted, and about the use of medications and other treatment procedures, specially designed literature can be useful and is a valuable adjunct to counselling. It is important to ensure that written information is comprehensible to the patient and to the relatives. Much of the health literature in use in rehabilitation programmes is of little value because it is poorly understood by patients, and particularly by the less well educated (Conroy & Mulcahy 1985).

PROGNOSIS AND RISK STRATIFICATION

An accurate prognosis is essential at the time of discharge from hospital if we hope to plan an appropriate exercise and rehabilitation programme for our patients. This is best done by a process of risk stratification designed to assess subsequent morbidity and mortality. While left ventricular function may be the greatest determinant of prognosis, other significant prognostic factors must be considered. However, left ventricular function is a particularly important deciding factor in relation to the type of exercise we may prescribe, particularly in the early stages of rehabilitation. There is now strong if not compelling evidence that regular aerobic exercise makes an independent contribution to improved survival in post-myocardial infarction patients (Oldrige et al 1988) but there is also some, but less convincing, evidence that improved survival is counterbalanced by a higher non-fatal myocardial infarction incidence in the active patients (Blackburn & Jacobs 1988). The risk of a subsequent non-fatal event may be higher in the early stages of convalescence and in the patient with significant heart muscle damage. It is important, therefore, to proceed cautiously with graduated exercises in the patient with significant heart muscle damage, not only to avoid early complications but also to permit adequate and sufficient time for the damaged myocardium to undergo healing and to recover optimum function.

An accurate and practical estimate of left ventricular function can be made from careful clinical evaluation. A history of recent or past left ventricular failure, dependency on inotropic drugs, clinical or radiological cardiomegaly, a poor exercise capacity in the absence of significant pulmonary disease, a persistent third heart sound or sinus tachycardia, a propensity to supraventricular or ventricular arrhythmias, and extensive changes in the ECG will point to significant and often severe impairment of left ventricular function. These findings will also convince the physician of the need for longterm inotropic support and for prudence in designing an aerobic exercise programme.

A submaximal exercise ECG, either before discharge or early in the course of convalescence, is now frequently advocated and employed to measure left ventricular function and exercise capacity (Fioretti et al 1987). In some centres the exercise test is now routinely employed in the early stages in most post-infarction patients. While the safety of early exercise testing has been established, it is not an essential adjunct to practical clinical assessment of left ventricular function (Cleempoel et al 1988).

Left ventricular wall motion, ejection fraction, and resting end diastolic pressure are also measured by echocardiography, nucleotide (MUGA) and ventriculography studies. These tests of left ventricular function may be useful in exceptional cases, when clinical findings are equivocal, but they lack the high degree of sensitivity and specificity which would render them a necessary addition to clinical evaluation.

Early angiography may be indicated in patients with post-infarction angina, particularly with some left ventricular impairment, and in certain other circumstances. The decision to perform angiography is not an easy one and may have important implications for the patient in terms of over-stressing the need for surgery. Useful guidelines have been laid down to assist us in deciding the need for angiography and should be adhered to (Ross et al 1987, 1989). Persistent post-infarction angina of effort or unstable angina, and marked ischaemic changes in the exercise stress test, are important indications for angiography.

While caution is advocated in prescribing early exercise programmes for patients with extensive left ventricular damage, experience has shown that, even in such patients, a useful training effect can be achieved by an appropriate programme (Squires et al 1987, Arvan 1988). It is seldom that the committed rehabilitation physician or team needs to prescribe a sedentary life for post-myocardial infarction patients, and then only in those with persistent congestive failure or near end-stage disease. It is also apparent that the adverse prognosis in patients with extensive myocardial damage is largely confined to the first year or two after the acute event, and that, having survived the early years, the prognosis reverts closely to that of patients with less extensive lesions (Weinblatt et al 1968). By appropriate graduated steps, these patients can successfully undertake regular symptom-limited exercise without added hazard.

Apart from left ventricular function, other adverse prognostic factors must be considered in risk stratification after myocardial infarction:

1. Increasing age
2. Previous angina
3. Frequent or multifocal ventricular ectopic beats or ventricular rhythms
4. Other vascular disease
5. Diabetes mellitus
6. Poorly controlled hypertension
7. Persistent hypotension
8. Persistent hyperlipidaemia
9. Continued smoking

10. Obesity
11. Concomitant systemic disease
12. Poor compliance to medication and risk factor modification
13. Poor social circumstances.

The presence of one or more of these added factors need not discourage active rehabilitation but may underline the need for special attention to medical or psychological problems, and may stress the importance of risk factor modification and behaviourial changes. They may also underline the need for special family and social support.

While treatment of hyperlipidaemia and hypertension as secondary prevention measures has not yet been convincingly shown to improve prognosis, such measures are justified on rational grounds, and in reducing other vascular and non-vascular complications. The effect of stopping smoking has been widely confirmed, with a reduced subsequent mortality of 25-50% reported from several centres (Mulcahy 1983).

REFERENCES

Arvan S 1988 Exercise performance of the high risk acute myocardial infarction patient after cardiac rehabilitation. American Journal of Cardiology 62:197-201

Blackburn H, Jacobs D R Jr 1988 Physical activity and the risk of coronary heart disease. New England Journal of Medicine 312:1217-1219

Cleempoel H, Vainsel H, Dramaix M et al 1988 Limitations on the prognostic value of predischarge data after myocardial infarction. British Heart Journal 60:98-103

Conroy M, Mulcahy R 1985 Readability of literature written for cardiac patients. Clinical Cardiology 8:104-106

Fioretti P, Tijssen J G, Azaar A R et al 1987 Prognostic value of predischarge 12 lead electrocardiogram after myocardial infarction compared with other routine clinical variables. British Heart Journal 57:306-312

Mulcahy R 1983 Influence of cigarette smoking on morbidity and mortality after myocardial infarction. British Heart Journal 49:410-415

Oldridge N B, Guyatt G H, Fischer M E, Rimm A A 1988 Cardiac rehabilitation after myocardial infarction. Combined experience of randomized clinical trials. Journal of the American Medical Association 260:945-950

Ross J Jr, Brandenburg R O, Dinsmore R E et al 1987 Guidelines for coronary angiography: report of the Joint American College of Cardiology/American Heart Association Task Force on Assessment of Cardiovascular Procedures. Journal American College of Cardiology 10:935-950 and Circulation 76:A963-977

Ross J Jr, Gilpin E A, Madsen E B et al 1989 A decision scheme for coronary angiography after acute myocardial infarction. Circulation 79:292-303

Squires R W, Lavie C J, Brandt T R, Gau G T, Bailey K R 1987 Cardiac rehabilitation in patients with severe ischaemic left ventricular dysfunction. Mayo Clinic Proceedings 62:997-1002

Weinblatt E, Shapiro S, Frank C W, Sager R V 1968 Prognosis of men after first myocardial infarction: mortality and first recurrence in relation to select parameters. American Journal of Public Health 58:1329-1347

FURTHER READING

Fardy P S, Yanowitz F G, Wilson P K (eds) 1988 Cardiac Rehabilitation, Adult Fitness, and Exercise Testing. Lea and Febiger, Philadelphia, 2nd edition

Hall L K, Meyer G C, Hellestein H K (eds) 1984 Cardiac Rehabilitation: Exercise Testing and Prescription. LaCross Exercise and Health Series

Hall L K, Meyer G F (eds) 1988 Cardiac Rehabilitation: Exercise Testing and Prescription Vol 11. LaCross Exercise and Health Series

Kellermann J J (ed) 1982 Comprehensive Cardiac Rehabilitation. Proceedings of the Second World Congress on Cardiac Rehabilitation. Advances in Cardiology 31:1-245

Wenger NK (ed) 1986 Rehabilitation: A Component of Comprehensive Cardiac Care. Bibliotheca Cardiologica 40:1-132

7. Treatment of symptoms and complications

There are certain specific symptoms and complications which we must anticipate, prevent and treat in patients who have recovered from myocardial infarction. The prevalence of post-infarction complications depends to a large extent on the degree of left ventricular damage and, to a lesser degree, on the extent and severity of disease of the coronary vessels.

ANGINA OF EFFORT

Angina of effort occurs in about 25% of patients after a first infarction and is most frequent in those with pre-infarction angina. It can vary in severity in some patients from time to time, depending on behavioural, therapeutic, circumstantial, climatic and seasonal factors. Angina is not a contraindication to achieving full recovery and a return to a normal life, but it may be a source of disability if it is sufficiently severe to reduce the patient's exercise capacity. If angina is mild and non-disabling, it may simply be a means of preventing a patient adopting too vigorous or sustained an exercise programme.

Patients with angina of effort following myocardial infarction usually have significant three vessel disease but the extent of heart damage may vary. Exercise testing will be indicated and may be helpful in delineating the extent, degree and location of the ischaemic myocardium, and thus in quantifying the severity of the disease. It is an essential procedure in most patients before a decision is taken to perform a coronary angiogram and to consider coronary artery surgery or angioplasty. However, the exercise test may be unhelpful in confirming the diagnosis of angina and in delineating the extent of the ischaemia if there are abnormalities in the resting ECG or if the patient is unable or unwilling to perform the test properly. A thallium 201 exercise ECG will be most useful if the ischaemic changes are difficult to interpret during and after exercise, and a pyridamole exercise test or atrial pacing may be required when the patient is unable to perform the exercise test. However, the value of these latter tests in decision making is open to considerable doubt.

Angioplasty and surgery may be indicated in post-infarction angina or in unstable angina, but many patients are not suitable because of unfavourable coronary morphology, poor left ventricular function, or refusal to submit to surgery. Many others do not require such intervention if they are favourable candidates for risk factor modification. There is still much we can do for patients by a conservative approach, including risk factor intervention, graduated exercise programmes, and using anti-anginal drugs. Angina of effort should not be regarded as an adverse and disabling complication but as a challenge and a measure of response to rehabilitation measures. A programme of graduated aerobic exercise, combined with strict risk-factor intervention in relation to smoking, hypertension and hyperlipidaemia, adequate weight reduction in the obese, and the use of anti-anginal drugs, has been successful in reducing the severity of angina in most of our post-myocardial infarction patients. Some patients become angina-free for long periods or permanently, and they can often dispense with the use of drugs as their symptoms become less obtrusive. It is not generally realised that angina can vary considerably in severity and frequency in post-myocardial infarction patients treated along these lines. Our own experience testifies to the value of such a conservative approach (Daly et al 1986).

Beta-blockers and calcium antagonists are recommended to reduce the severity of angina and to increase the patient's exercise tolerance. However, in our experience, sublingual nitrates or a nitrate spray have proved to be most useful in preventing anticipated pain or in relieving pain when it occurs. Patients should be carefully instructed in the use of nitrates. When properly used, nitrates greatly facilitate exercise performance and contribute to an improved cardiac and peripheral training effect. It is a useful measure of progress to keep a record of the quantity of nitrates used and to relate consumption with the intensity of the patient's exercise programme. Nitrates, beta-blockers and calcium antagonists need not be continued indefinitely. When the patient is no longer troubled by symptoms, a gradual reduction of drugs with eventual withdrawal can be achieved.

Patients and their relatives should be familiar with the nature of cardiac pain, and should be instructed to differentiate it from pain of non-cardiac origin. The recognition of cardiac pain will alert the patient who presents with crescendo or unstable angina, so that early professional advice can be sought.

LEFT VENTRICULAR FAILURE AND CONGESTIVE HEART FAILURE

Most patients admitted with acute left ventricular failure to hospital emergency departments in western countries today will be found to have had a fresh or previous myocardial infarction, with significant heart muscle damage. Hypertensive heart disease and aortic valve disease are now less common causes of left ventricular failure, as are cardiomyopathies and other less common cardiopathies. Proper assessment of left ventricular function before discharge should alert us to this risk. Left ventricular function assessment is dealt with in some detail in Chapter 6 page 51. In patients perceived to have significant left ventricular damage after infarction, the need for subsequent interrupted or regular diuretic treatment may be indicated. Some physicians would also prescribe maintenance digitalis therapy. Patients should be advised to take note of increasing dyspnoea on effort or of mild orthopnoea, when diuretic therapy may also be tried. Care should be taken to avoid precipitating causes of left ventricular failure, such as excessively vigorous exercise or severe avoidable emotional situations. Respiratory infections may also precipitate heart failure in susceptible subjects and certain drugs with a negatively inotropic effect, such as the non-steroidal analgesics and beta-blockers, should be prescribed with caution.

Congestive heart failure, manifested by fatigue, dyspnoea, hepatic engorgement, dependent oedema and raised venous pressure, will need inotropic support, including diuretics and possibly digitalis, peripheral vasodilators and ACE inhibitors. Exercise may be contra-indicated in these patients, and the presence of congestive failure may be an indication of an advanced ischaemic cardiomyopathy. There may, however, be a precipitating cause, such as the recent onset of rapid atrial fibrillation or a respiratory infection. In such an event the elimination or treatment of the precipitating cause may be effective.

ARRHYTHMIAS

Supraventricular arrhythmias, particularly atrial fibrillation and flutter, and paroxysmal atrial tachycardia, are not uncommon in post-myocardial infarction patients and after heart surgery. Electrical or medical cardioversion, with quinidine for atrial fibrillation and atrial flutter, may be justified if the arrhythmia is of recent onset and if there is not severe heart muscle damage. Intravenous verapamil will be effective in paroxysmal tachycardia. Otherwise these patients with persistent or recurring arrhythmias are best treated by maintenance digitalis in appropriate doses. Some physicians will favour the addition of longterm anticoagulant treatment to reduce risk of thrombo-embolism, particularly in the presence of congestive failure or a history of previous embolism.

Ventricular ectopic rhythms are the rule in post-myocardial infarction patients, when monitored by continuous Holter recordings. They are usually asymptomatic but may be symptomatic, particularly in anxious patients and in those with extensive heart muscle damage. Continuous monitoring may reveal ectopic rhythms extending from occasional or frequent unifocal ectopics, occasional or frequent couplets, triplets, or salvoes of ectopics, multifocal ectopics, and ventricular tachycardia. Ventricular tachycardia may vary from occasional short-lived asymptomatic bouts to prolonged symptomatic and life-threatening tachyarrhythmias. The correct management of ventricular arrhythmias is still a source of uncertainty and of controversy, because their prognostic significance is often far from clear, except in the case of unifocal right ventricular ectopics, when they are of little significance, and in the case of symptomatic ventricular tachycardia, when they may be of grave prognostic importance. The value of the anti-arrhythmic drugs in prevention and treatment is also far from clear, and indeed some drugs may aggravate the arrhythmic tendency and may adversely affect left ventricular function through negatively-intropic mechanisms. Torsade de Points, or reciprocating ventricular fibrillation, is one life-threatening arrhythmia which may be provoked by anti-arrhythmic drugs, such as disopyramide or mexiletine.

Asymptomatic ventricular ectopic rhythms, such as unifocal ectopics in singles, couplets or triplets, and multifocal ectopics or asymptomatic bouts of ventricular tachycardia, should not be prescribed specific anti-arrhythmic drugs, but underlying precipitating causes, such as poor left ventricular function, early decompensation, recurring ischaemia, and disorders of electrolytes should be sought and remedied. Symptomatic, and possibly complex, ventricular rhythms are best treated with one of the recognised anti-arrhythmic drugs, such as disopyramide, mexiletine, quinine or perhexiline. Treatment is best conducted under cardiological supervision. A trial and error approach may be required. If electrophysiology studies are available, it may be possible to identify the appropriate anti-arrhythmic drugs through such studies, and, in some persistent life-threatening situations, it may be possible to inactivate the offending part of the myocardium through fulguration or a resection of the arrhythmogenic focus, although the reported mortality after surgery may be significant (Cox 1983). However, results of surgical intervention now appear to be improving.

In practice, serious life-threatening ventricular arrhythmias not responding to elimination of a precipitating cause or to conventional drug therapy, respond best to amiodarone. Despite a high propensity to side-effects, this drug has proved safe and highly effective in our hands, subject to careful monitoring and titration of dosage. It is not significantly negatively inotropic, unlike other anti-arrhythmic preparations, and therefore is unlikely to precipitate heart failure in susceptible subjects. It may in a few cases induce Torsade de Points. A satisfactory maintenance dose is about 200mg daily.

HEART BLOCK AND BRADYARRHYTHMIAS

The different manifestations of heart block may require attention during the rehabilitation period. Right or left bundle branch block is usually a complication of ischaemia during the acute stage and does not normally persist after recovery. If persistent, bundle branch block may have been present previous to the attack or may indicate significant heart damage. It requires no specific treatment, apart from attention to possible left ventricular dysfunction.

Bifascicular or trifascicular block implies interference with one or two of the three fasciculi extending from the bundle of His, with or without delayed atrioventricular transmission. The patient may be at risk of complete atrioventricular dissociation, which may lead to irreversible and fatal asystole. In the presence of significant symptoms, such as syncope or dizzy attacks, permanent pacing is obligatory. A cardiological opinion should be sought in patients with bifascicular or trifascicular block. Atrioventricular dissociation in its various manifestations of first, second and third degree block, is a common complication during the acute stage and has an unfavourable prognostic significance. However, it commonly reverts to normal conduction if the patient survives the acute stage. Persistence of first degree block certainly merits observation and repeated Holter monitoring. If the patient is complaining of dizzy episodes, syncope or convulsions, it requires permanent pacing. Persistent or intermittent second or third degree block is best treated by permanent pacing, but there may be exceptions to this course. The opinion of a cardiologist should be sought in this situation.

Sino-atrial disease may be encountered in patients with coronary heart disease. It is not uncommon in older people who are otherwise apparently healthy. It is also common in chronic respiratory disease. It is manifested by irregular sino-atrial discharge, by abnormal p-wave morphology in the ECG and, in symptomatic patients, by tachyarrhythmias or bradyarrhythmias or, not uncommonly, both. Tachyarrhythmias may be successfully treated with digitalis or other anti-arrhythmic agents but such treatment not infrequently unmasks or aggravates the tendency to symptomatic bradyarrhythmias. In this situation, permanent pacing with the use of drugs to control tachyarrhythmias is the treatment of choice.

REFERENCES

Cox J L 1983 Surgery for cardiac arrhythmias. Current Problems in Cardiology 8: 1-60

Daly L E, Hickey N, Mulcahy R 1986 Course of angina pectoris after an acute coronary event. British Medical Journal 293:653-656

8. Prevention of morbidity and early mortality

A considerable amount of attention has been paid to the need to reduce the risk of infarction and its consequences during the acute stage of unstable angina, and to reduce the risk of extension or recurrence of infarction during the acute stage of myocardial infarction. Attention has also been directed to reducing risk of subsequent coronary morbidity and mortality in patients who suffer from angina of effort or who have recovered from unstable angina or myocardial infarction, or from coronary artery surgery.

Attempts at reducing the risk of further morbidity and mortality include the elimination of risk factors, exercise programmes, the use of drugs, surgery or angioplasty. These will be dealt with in separate sections. While we must acknowledge the importance of the current approach to preventing or reducing the extent of infarction during the acute stage, the purpose of this monograph on rehabilitation is to direct attention to longterm attempts to prevent recurring coronary events as well as other vascular and non-vascular complications and mortality. Reducing risk of further coronary and non-coronary events is one of the principal objectives of longterm management of coronary patients. It not only contributes to health and longevity, but should enhance the subject's quality of life, and, in our experience, makes a major contribution to a reduction in anxiety and depression as patients perceive the purpose of these interventions.

DRUGS

Several trials have reported the effect of drugs in preventing or reducing the extent of myocardial infarction in the coronary care unit. Nitrates, beta-blockers and calcium antagonists are widely used in the management of unstable angina, not only for the purpose of alleviating symptoms, but also allegedly to reduce the risk of infarction and death. Despite the widespread use of these drugs, often described as 'maximum medical therapy', there is little evidence in the literature to justify their use as agents in improving immediate prognosis. They may be of value in reducing the severity of rest pain but nitrates in their various forms, whether inhaled, sublingual, transdermal or intravenous, are the most flexible and effective for this purpose. A criticism of the conventional drug treatment of unstable angina has been presented (Mulcahy et al 1985, Mulcahy 1990).

There have been a number of trials which have reported on the influence of beta-blockers, aspirin, anticoagulants and calcium antagonists on immediate prognosis in patients with acute myocardial infarction (Yosuf et al 1988). Some trials have shown benefit in terms of improved early mortality. However, other trials have reported negative results (Yosuf et al 1988) and there are a number of inconsistencies in terms of the drugs used, their dosage, the age group of the patients, the nature, location and extent of the infarction, the comparability of the trials and the end-points assessed. It is significant that, despite the advocacy of drugs specifically prescribed to improve survival during the acute stage, controversy still exists, disagreements of benefit continue, and cardiologists and physicians vary widely in their acceptance of the benefit of these drugs. The advocacy of anticoagulant drugs during the acute stage has continued for more than 30 years. Anticoagulant therapy has been largely rejected by the profession, but we are still reminded from time to time by the few protagonists of its value. The advocacy of beta-blockers and calcium antagonists in the management of unstable angina has continued for 20 years or more, but they still remain of unproven value (Mulcahy et al 1985, Mulcahy 1990). Recently, the use of intravenous thrombolytic agents provide the best means of improving prognosis at the earlier acute stage (ISIS-2 Trial 1988).

A number of trials have claimed that medication commenced during or immediately after the acute stage and continued for defined periods after recovery may beneficially influence later morbidity and mortality in terms of reducing further coronary events and life-threatening arrhythmias. Aspirin in the management of unstable angina, and beta-blockers in the longterm management of unstable angina and myocardial infarction have been advocated on the basis of several trials. Calcium antagonists, dipyridamole, sulphinpyrazone (Antiplatelet Trial 1988, Fitzgerald 1987) and other drugs have been advocated but without convincing evidence. The ISIS-2 trial involving 17,000 patients with acute myocardial infarction showed considerable benefit in terms of reduced coronary mortality and non-fatal myocardial infarction in patients treated with aspirin and with aspirin and thrombolysis during the acute stage (ISIS-2 Trial 1988).

A number of trials have reported benefit in terms of improved prognosis with longterm beta-blocker therapy after infarction (Yosuf et al 1988). However, the compelling significance of these trials has not been accepted by many physicians. This can be attributed to a number of inconsistencies, including negative results reported from a number of trials, varying benefits in terms of age of patients, location of infarct, size of infarction, the presence of certain risk factors, such as smoking, dosage and type of beta-blocker, the mode of death, and the date of commencement of treatment in relation to the initial event. A further difficulty in adopting routine beta-blocker therapy is based on the type of patients included in the trials, the exclusion factors and the difficulty of relating the trials' exclusion factors to treatment of one's acute coronary patients. In looking objectively at the evidence supporting the use of beta-blockers after recovery from myocardial infarction, it is not possible to give clear guidelines about their use. The decision about their use must be left to the individual physician, who must balance the apparent benefits against the uncertainties in terms of cost and possible side effects of the drugs, not to mention the possible adverse psychological effects of longterm medication on patients who should be encouraged to return to a normal life.

In summary, clear guidelines cannot at present be given about the advisability of prescribing medication for every patient with the specific purpose of reducing the risk of further coronary events. This conclusion does not of course refer to drugs used in the control of hypertension, hyperlipidaemia, diabetes and other risk factors, which may prevent cardiac and non-cardiac complications, and which may contribute to reducing mortality. Drugs may adversely affect quality of life through their side effects. These side effects may not be of serious significance or too obtrusive, but the patient's well-being may improve when medication is terminated. Drugs are a reminder of the patient's illness and dependency, and may thus have an adverse psychological effect. For these reasons we should ensure that the advantages of drugs exceed their disadvantages before prescribing longterm therapy.

SURGERY AND ANGIOPLASTY

A minority of patients with coronary heart disease will benefit by coronary artery surgery or by angioplasty. These procedures may be indicated during the acute stage, particularly in patients with unstable angina and persistent rest pain, but there is still considerable uncertainty about their advantages at this stage over a conservative medical approach.

Coronary artery surgery and angioplasty may be needed during the early or late convalescent stage for the purpose of relieving unstable angina and disabling angina of effort, and, by reducing the risk of further coronary events, to improve life expectation. It is doubtful if coronary artery surgery has a place in improving chronic left ventricular dysfunction (Bounous et al 1988), nor is there evidence of benefit in patients with persistent life-threatening ventricular arrhythmias, except perhaps when they are associated with acute ischaemic episodes.

While there is little disagreement about the efficacy of coronary artery surgery in reducing the symptoms of chronic angina, at least in most patients for an appreciable period which may be measured in years, and in terminating the rest pain of unstable angina, there is less evidence to support the contention of an improved life expectation, except in patients with left main stem or main stem equivalent disease, and in those with moderately impaired left ventricular function and three vessel disease (Killip et al 1985). While the design of these studies leaves much to be desired in terms of comparability of surgical and non-surgical groups, and because of cross-over problems, it is now an acceptable part of rehabilitation and longterm management to consider symptomatic patients as potential candidates for coronary surgery or angioplasty.

Angioplasty has been widely adopted in recent years and appears to be a relatively safe procedure, with good results in terms of symptomatic relief, at least over the short term, in experienced hands (Baim 1988). With experience and improved techniques, a wider selection of patients may be considered for this procedure. There is as yet no evidence to suggest improved prognosis and life expectation in patients subjected to angioplasty, nor are we likely to have clear answers to this question unless properly designed controlled studies are carried out. So far such studies have not been reported. Most studies of the results of angioplasty report benefit in terms of pain relief of 50-80%, with a substantial minority who derive no benefit, and with 2-5% who may develop fatal arrhythmias, or fatal or non-fatal infarction, during the procedure or who may require emergency coronary artery surgery. There is also a substantial minority who suffer early recurrence of symptoms, requiring repeat angioplasty, coronary artery surgery or a decision to treat the patient by conservative means (Baim 1988).

In conclusion, coronary artery surgery and angioplasty have a role in the rehabilitation and longterm management of selected patients. The availability of these treatment modalities does, however, present us with certain imponderables, such as the indications for surgery in asymptomatic patients, when a decision to operate is based on an anatomical rather than a functional assessment of the coronary arteriogram, and where improvement in survival is a doubtful consequence. It is likely that many of these patients do not benefit from surgery, that the decision to operate is based on too limited a view of the benefits of comprehensive conservative treatment, and on exaggerated perceptions of the benefits of surgery. Careful judgement is necessary before committing patients to surgical intervention. The availability of an independent second opinion would reduce the number of patients who are subjected to surgery without adequate reasons. These recommendations are compellingly made in an editorial in the Journal of the American Medical Association (Mulley & Eagle 1988).

It is imperative that patients undergoing surgery or angioplasty should be well informed about the nature, indications and likely benefits of these procedures. Like survivors of myocardial infarction, they require full rehabilitation support subsequently. This applies particularly to intervention in relation to smoking, hyperlipidaemia and hypertension control, because of the vulnerability of the grafts to atherosclerotic changes and to thrombosis (Campeau et al 1984, Dion et al 1982). The special rehabilitation problems and requirements of post-surgical patients are referred to in Chapter 16.

REFERENCES

Antiplatelet Trial 1988 Antiplatelet Trialists Collaboration. Secondary prevention of vascular disease by prolonged antiplatelet treatment. British Medical Journal 296:320-331

Baim D S 1988 In: E Braunwald (ed) Heart disease: a text book of cardiovascular medicine (3rd edition). W B Saunders & Co, Philadelphia, pp 1379-1389

Bounous E P, Mark D B, Pollock B G et al 1988 Surgical survival benefits for coronary disease patients with left ventricular dysfunction. Circulation 78:1151-1157

Campeau, L, Enjalbert M, Lesperance J et al 1984 The relation of risk factors to the development of atherosclerosis in saphenous-vein bypass grafts and the progression of disease in the native circulation. A study 10 years after aortocoronary bypass surgery. New England Journal of Medicine 311:1329-1332

Dion W F, Grevenow P, Pollock M L et al 1982 Medical problems and physiologic responses during supervised inpatient cardiac rehabilitation: the patient after coronary artery bypass grafting. Heart and Lung 11:248-255

Fitzgerald G A 1987 Dipyridamole. New England Journal of Medicine 316:1247-1257 and 317:1734-1736

ISIS-2 Trial 1988 Randomized trial of intravenous streptokinase, oral aspirin, both, or neither among 17,187 cases of suspected acute myocardial infarction: ISIS-2 Collaborative Group. Lancet 2:349-360

Killip T, Passamani E, Davis K, CASS 1985 Coronary artery surgery study (CASS): a randomized trial of coronary bypass surgery: eight years follow-up and survival in patients with reduced ejection fraction. Circulation 72:V102-109

Mulcahy R 1990 Does intensive medical therapy influence the outcome of unstable angina? Clinical Cardiology (in press)

Mulcahy R, Al Awadhi A H, De Buitleir M, Tobin G, Johnson H, Conroy R 1985 Natural History and prognosis of unstable angina. American Heart Journal 109:753-758

Mulley Jr A G, Eagle K M 1988 What is inappropriate care? Journal of the American Medical Association 260 (editorial): 540-541

Yosuf S, Wittes J, Friedman L 1988 Overview of results of randomized clinical trials in heart disease I. Treatments following myocardial infarction. Journal of the American Medical Association 260:2088-2093

SECTION 3

Secondary Prevention

9. Risk factor intervention and behaviour modification

The importance of risk factor intervention as part of rehabilitation and secondary prevention was not fully appreciated in the past but it is now receiving greater attention as an integral part of good management. Risk factor intervention receives less attention from clinicians than treatment modalities based on drugs and surgical intervention, and frequently is not included in recommendations about longterm management. Such an omission leaves a serious gap in our approach to the needs of patients suffering from a progressive disease, the causes of which are now largely known. Apart from the limited evidence from trials supporting the value of risk factor identification and elimination, there is an inherent logic and an obvious rationale in identifying all possible atherogenic and thrombogenic agents, and of attempting to retard or stop the progress of the underlying disease.

Advantages derived from risk factor intervention include a reduced incidence of subsequent fatal and non-fatal coronary events, and of post-infarction angina and heart failure. We can anticipate less frequent occlusion of coronary grafts, and less risk of advancing peripheral vascular disease, stroke or aneurysm. Non-vascular conditions such as chronic respiratory diseases will also benefit. Anxiety about further coronary events, including sudden death, is alleviated when patients perceive the logic of eliminating the cause or causes of the underlying disease.

Assiduous risk factor elimination and control may be the single most important step in successful rehabilitation and in improving survival. Control must be global in that all possible adverse factors should be identified and eliminated. Only one randomised trial testifies to the benefits of a global approach in terms of mortality and sudden death (Hamalainen et al 1989), but there is supporting evidence from the meta-analysis of 14 randomised controlled trials of exercise and secondary prevention programmes reported by Oldridge et al (1988).

There are inherent problems in the execution and design of trials which make it difficult to reach unequivocal conclusions about the benefits of a global risk factor approach. The benefits of stopping smoking in relation to the prevention of post-infarction angina, and in reducing non-fatal and particularly fatal myocardial infarction and sudden death, have been firmly established (Mulcahy 1983). The control of hypertension (Graham et al 1978, Connolly et al 1983) and hyperlipidaemia (Canner et al 1986) has shown benefit according to some reports, but trials of secondary prevention have been inadequate, so that hypertension and hyperlipidaemia control rest on tenuous evidence of benefit. In advocating control of hypertension and hyperlipidaemia, we are relying on the assumption that our intervention will slow the process of atherogenesis and reduce the risk of non-coronary hypertensive complications. There is evidence from animal and human studies that strict reduction of saturated fat and cholesterol intake, with or without chemotherapy, aimed at normalising the lipid profile, will lead to the arrest or regression of atherogenesis (Arntzenius et al 1985, Blankenhorn et al 1978, 1987, 1988, Brensike et al 1984, Duffield et al 1983, Nash et al 1984, Nikkila et al 1984)

Obesity is not an established independent risk factor for coronary heart disease but its control is advised because of its role as a non-specific risk factor for health and longevity. Diabetes mellitus requires diligent control in the coronary patient as in any other victim of this condition, and other vascular and non-vascular conditions need to be identified and treated as indicated.

LONGTERM COMPLIANCE

The importance of risk factor identification and intervention needs to be stressed from the earliest stages and soon after admission to coronary care. Apart from routine counselling, appropriate literature will be helpful in educating the patient and family members. All members of the cardiac team should be familiar with the evidence implicating the principal risk factors of hyperlipidaemia, hypertension and smoking, and should be capable of discussing this evidence and of giving guidance about necessary changes in life-style and behaviour. Group sessions, to which family members are invited, are useful for an exchange of information and to identify problems patients may have in adhering to appropriate advice. Early adherence to dietary, exercise and smoking advice may be satisfactory because of the recent perception of a life-threatening illness and the close contact with the cardiac team and with other patients. However, longterm compliance with life-style changes may create major problems in the absence of repeated counselling and medical supervision. Perhaps the greatest single failing in cardiac rehabilitation remains the record of poor compliance with smoking control, dietary advice, aerobic exercise, and alcohol limitation, which is reported from the longterm studies which are available (German 1988). Only by providing longterm supervision at a rehabilitation and secondary prevention clinic, or by regular supervision by general practitioners who are adequately trained in patient counselling, can any substantial improvement be achieved in encouraging patients to adhere to desirable behaviourial changes.

We have encouraged all patients under 60 years seen by us since 1961, who have suffered an initial myocardial infarction, to attend a rehabilitation and secondary prevention clinic annually, after more frequent visits during the first two years following the initial event. About 1750 patients were invited to attend regularly from 1961 to 1985. This arrangement created no serious logistic problems for our small rehabilitation group, all of whom are members of the cardiac team. Two outpatient sessions per week were sufficient to deal with these and other patients. We have reported return to work rates consistently around 90% since 1966 (Mulcahy et al 1988). We have also reported compliance with exercise programmes two years after the initial event in about 50% of patients who had been sedentary beforehand (Mulcahy 1985) and cessation of smoking at the end of two years in 70% of initial smokers (Hickey et al 1981). We believe these relatively satisfactory results can be attributed to annual supervision and re-inforcement of advice by the cardiac team, including the cardiologists who attended the patients in coronary care.

Patient and family involvement

Patients and family members should be encouraged to become involved in their own management in certain areas. Hypertensive patients are instructed to monitor their own blood pressure and in some cases to titrate their drug treatment according to their blood pressure response (Fitzgerald et al 1985). Self-monitoring of blood pressure makes an important contribution to the patient's understanding of blood pressure control. Control is improved through better compliance with medication and non-pharmacological measures and this control frequently extends to other behavioural changes. Maintaining the necessary life-style changes poses one of the greatest problems in longterm management of patients. Reverting to old life-style habits occurs too readily, when the crisis is deemed to be past, when the patient has returned to good health, when 'the tear is no longer in the eye'. There has been insufficient attention to this aspect of coronary rehabilitation and no amount of counselling or encouragement will achieve success without constant reinforcement of advice, at least for the first two or three years after myocardial infarction or surgery.

The success rate of the various behavioural changes which may be recommended differs widely according to the nature of the advice, the feasibility of its adoption and the motivation of the patient. Longterm adherence to weight control and exercise programmes tends to be poor, while smoking cessation and dietary change aimed at hyperlipidaemia control are reasonably satisfactory. Smoking cessation is particularly good if the patient stops smoking immediately and does not resume in the early days of convalescence. In our experience, patients who achieve a major reduction in smoking but do not stop completely have a poor record, with recidivism in about 80% at the end of one year. Treatment among hypertensives and diabetics is seen to be satisfactory for the great majority, a fact which we attribute to patient and family involvement in management and to the partnership which exists between patient, spouse, family doctor and the rehabilitation team.

The influence of social class

Educational and occupational class play a role in determining compliance with life-style changes, with the better educated showing sustained response to smoking cessation, exercise programme and early return to work (Conroy et al 1986). These differences can be explained, at least partly, by the educated person's better response to health education and to the understanding of the health message, and by his or her cultural background which encourages a more flexible and innovative approach to life-style change. The less educated are not necessarily immune to health education and advice, but they require a more sustained effort to achieve success and this requires repeated reinforcement. The written word and the written message are less easily understood by the less educated (Conroy & Mulcahy 1985). We need to employ alternative methods, perhaps through visual or anecdotal means, or through group sessions and peer example, to achieve better results. Industrial health programmes conducted at the worksite hold a special promise in dealing with the less educated.

Factors influencing compliance

The following factors play an important role in achieving satisfactory longterm compliance with desirable behavioural changes in coronary patients:

* Well informed, repeated advice and education to stress the scientific basis of risk factor identification and modification
* Counselling by verbal means on a one-to-one basis, as well as through group sessions. Health literature should be available to reinforce counselling

* Longterm supervision, at least for one to two years, to reinforce advice, to supervise programmes, and to provide fresh guidance about physical and psychosocial capabilities
* Patient and family involvement in management; encourage family and social support
* Appropriate life-style changes should be encouraged and supported. Attitudes implying criticism or moralising should be avoided, particularly by the spouse and the family members. Cautionary advice by family and family doctor should be discouraged
* Cognisance should be taken of the patients personality and moods. Type A behaviour may need modification and mood changes should respond to counselling, explanation and, in a few cases, appropriate psychotherapy and medication.

REFERENCES

Arntzenius A C, Kromhout D, Borth J D et al 1985 Diet, lipoproteins and the progression of coronary atherosclerosis. The Leiden Intervention Trial. New England Journal of Medicine 312:805-811

Blankenhorn D H, Brooks S H, Selzer R H, Barndt R Jr 1978 The rate of atherosclerosis change during treatment of hyperlipoproteinaemia. Circulation 57:355-361

Blankenhorn D H, Nessim S A, Johnson R L, Sanmario M E, Azen S P, Cashin-Hemphill L 1987 Beneficial effects of combined colestipol-niacin therapy on coronary atherosclerosis and coronary venous bypass grafts. Journal of the American Medical Association 257:3233-3240

Blankenhorn D H, Johnson R L, El Zein H A, Vailas L I 1988 Dietary fat influences human coronary lesion information. Circulation 78:89-96

Brensike J F, Levy R I, Kelsey S F et al 1984 Effects on therapy with cholestyramine on progression of coronary atherosclerosis: results of the NHLBI Type 11 Coronary Intervention Study. Circulation 69:313-324

Canner P L, Berger K G, Wenger N K et al 1986 Fifteen year mortality in Coronary Drug Project patients: long-term benefit with niacin. Journal of the American College of Cardiology 8:1245-1255

Connolly D C, Elveback L R, Oxman HA 1983 Coronary heart disease in residents of Rochester, Minnesota, 1950-1975 111. Effect of hypertension and its treatment on survival of patients with coronary artery disease. Mayo Clinical Proceedings 58:259-264

Conroy R M, Mulcahy R 1985 Readability of literature written for cardiac patients. Clinical Cardiology 8:104-106

Conroy R, Mulcahy R, Graham I, Reid V, Cahill S 1986 Prediction of patient response to risk factor modification advice after admission for unstable angina or myocardial infarction. Journal of Cardiopulmonary Rehabilitation 6:344-357

Duffield R G, Lewis B, Miller N E, Jamieson C W, Brunt J N, Colchester A C 1983 Treatment of hyperlipidaemia retards progression of symptomatic femoral atherosclerosis. A randomized controlled trial. Lancet 2:639-642

Fitzgerald D J, O'Calaghan W G, O'Brien E, Johnson H, Mulcahy R, Hickey N 1985 Home recording of blood pressure in the management of hypertension. Irish Medical Journal 78:216-218

German P S 1988 Compliance and chronic disease. Hypertension 11:1156-1160

Graham I M, Mulcahy R, Hickey N, Daly L 1978 Effect of hypertension and its treatment on progress after myocardial infarction. In: Hjalmarson H, Wilhelmsen L (eds) Acute and long-term medical management of myocardial infarction Lindgren Molndal, pp 270-284

Hamalainen H, Luurila O J, Kallio V, Knuts L-R, Arstila M, Hakkila J 1989 long-term reduction in sudden deaths after a multifactorial intervention programme in patients with myocardial infarction: 10 year results of a controlled investigation. European Heart Journal 10:55-62

Hickey N, Graham I, Kennedy C, Daly L, Mulcahy R 1981 Trends in response to anti-smoking advice in patients with coronary heart disease between 1961 and 1975. Irish Journal of Medical Science 150:262-264

MRFIT Group 1982 Multiple risk factor intervention trial: risk factor changes and mortality. Journal of the American Medical Association 248:1465-1477

Mulcahy R 1983 Influence of cigarette smoking on morbidity and mortality after myocardial infarction. British Heart Journal 49:410-415

Mulcahy R 1985 The virtues of physical activity in secondary prevention of coronary heart disease. Tromso seminar 'The good things of life' (unpublished)

Mulcahy R, Kennedy C, Conroy R 1988 The long-term work record for post-infarction patients subjected to an informal rehabilitation and secondary prevention programme. European Heart Journal 9:L84-88

Nash D T, Gensini G, Esente P 1984 The progression of coronary atherosclerosis. Journal of Cardiac Rehabilitation 4:21-26

Nikkila E A, Viikinkoski P, Valle M, Frick M H 1984 Prevention of progression of coronary atherosclerosis by treatment of hyperlipidaemia: a seven year prospective angiographic study. British Medical Journal 289:220-223

Ross J Jr, Gilpin E A, Madsen E B, et al 1989 A decision scheme for coronary angiography after acute myocardial infarction. Circulation 79:292-303

Oldridge N B, Guyatt G H, Fischer M E, Rimm A A 1988 Cardiac rehabilitation after myocardial infarction. Combined experience of randomized clinical trials. Journal of the American Medical Association 260:945-950

Wissler R W, Vesselinovitch D 1983 Combined effects of cholestyramine and probucal on regression of atherosclerosis in rhesus monkey aortas. Applied Pathology 1:89-96

FURTHER READING

Konig K, Denolin H, Dorossiev D (eds) 2nd edition 1983 Myocardial Infarction. How to prevent, How to Rehabilitate: Scientific Council on Rehabilitation of Cardiac Patients, International Society and Federation of Cardiology, Boehringer Mannheim

May G S, Eberlein K A, Furberg C D, Passamani E R, DeMet D L 1982 Secondary prevention after myocardial infarction: a review of long-term trials. Progress in Cardiovascular Diseases 24:331-351

Mulcahy R 1982 The secondary prevention of coronary heart disease. Das Medizinische Prisma 4:1-20

Pyorala K, Rapaport E, Konig K, Schettler G, Dmdiehm P (eds) 1984 Secondary prevention of coronary disease. Workshop of the International Society and Federation of Cardiology. Titisee, Tithieme Stuttgart

10. Cholesterol

Hyperlipidaemia plays a key role in the genesis of atherosclerosis and coronary artery disease. Epidemiological evidence of a close relationship between high dietary saturated fat intake, high mean cholesterol levels and a high incidence of coronary heart disease is consistent with the hypothesis that the mean population lipid level is the most accurate indication of community risk of coronary heart disease. Hypertension and cigarette smoking have also been identified as primary coronary risk factors but their independent contribution is apparent only in populations with a high fat intake and a high incidence of hyperlipidaemia. Hence in Japan, where cigarette smoking and high blood pressure are at least as prevalent as in western countries, and where cholesterol levels are low, the incidence of coronary heart disease has remained at exceptionally low levels.

There is evidence derived from secular changes in coronary mortality in populations, and from logistic function data derived from prospective studies of coronary heart disease, that a 1% fall in the cholesterol level of a community may presage a 2-3% fall in coronary mortality (NIH Consensus 1985). It is reasonable to assume that population intervention studies should achieve a corresponding fall in coronary mortality through dietary intervention and cholesterol reduction. The added effect of smoking cessation and better blood pressure control on mortality cannot be easily assessed but again it would be reasonable to anticipate an enhancement of the effect of cholesterol control on coronary heart disease mortality by these public health measures.

The case for lipid lowering

Most patients surviving a myocardial infarction will show some evidence of hyperlipidaemia. Case-history studies of coronary patients confirm that mean cholesterol levels are substantially and significantly higher in such patients than in the normal population (Mulcahy et al 1967, 1969). Whether the results of dietary and other hypolipidaemic interventions in primary prevention programmes can be extrapolated to secondary prevention studies is a moot question, particularly in view of the advanced vascular disease which can be anticipated in coronary patients. Trials of secondary prevention have been poorly designed and are defective in other respects. Five studies report non-significant benefits, and four report negative results (Ball et al 1965, Bierenbaum et al 1970, Hansen et al 1962, Kallio et al 1979, Leren 1970, Medical Research Council 1968, Morrison 1960, Phillips et al 1988, Rose et al 1965). They have failed to give us clear guidelines, but the limited information available to us, both from primary and secondary studies, and the relative ease and safety of dietary modification and the success of lowering lipid levels, would justify a careful evaluation of the lipid status of our patients, and appropriate dietary intervention. In the more severe and intractable hyperlipidaemias, interrupted or continuous chemotherapy may be justified.

In the British Regional Heart Study (Phillips et al 1988), it was shown that coronary patients with high lipid levels are more prone to recurrence of myocardial infarction or sudden death, supporting a policy of reducing cholesterol by diet or, if necessary, by medication. There is also evidence that patients subjected to coronary artery surgery with high levels of cholesterol are more prone to graft occlusion (Campeau et al 1984). Two trials of hypolipidaemic drugs confirm their value in lowering coronary morbidity and mortality in survivors of myocardial infarction (Canner et al 1986, Carlson & Rosenhammer 1988).

Studies of regression of atherosclerosis in animals confirm the benefit of lipid lowering (Wissler & Vesselinovitch 1983) and recent promising reports of retardation and regression of atherosclerosis in humans (Arntzenius et al 1985, Blankenhorn et al 1978, 1987, 1988, Brensike et al 1984, Duffield et al 1983, Nash et al 1984, Nikkila et al 1984) permit us to be optimistic about the value of lipid control in secondary prevention.

THE APPROACH TO HYPERLIPIDAEMIA CONTROL

A total non-fasting cholesterol estimation is sufficient to alert us to the presence of hyperlipidaemia in population screening programmes. The current wisdom relating to cut-off points between normal and abnormal levels now underlines the importance of achieving cholesterol levels below 5.2mmol/L (200mg%). The latest recommendations about normal levels are available from the National Cholesterol Programme of the National Heart Lung and Blood Institute (National Cholesterol Education Programme 1989) and the European Atherosclerosis Society (European Atherosclerosis Society 1988), and should be followed in preventive practice.

There are special considerations in relation to lipid control in secondary prevention. The total cholesterol level, like other metabolic parameters, may be acutely and substantially reduced immediately after a myocardial infarction, with a fall in total cholesterol commencing during the first 24 hours, reaching its nadir about a week later, and returning to pre-myocardial infarction levels within a few weeks or months. The magnitude and duration of the decline is a measure of the size of the infarct.

We routinely perform a non-fasting cholesterol and HDL measurement in patients with confirmed or suspected coronary heart disease in our emergency department, but if such a result is not available, we attempt to estimate the pre-infarct cholesterol level by measuring the delay between the onset of the attack and the performance of the test, and by a clinical and enzyme assessment of infarct size.

The routine cholesterol level is a good general measure of hyperlipidaemia because it is an accurate measure of the common polygenic type of lipid disturbance, and of the less common heterozygous and homozygous types 2A and 2B hyperlipidaemias. The less common type 3 and type 4 hyperlipidaemias, where high triglyceride levels predominate, must be sought even in the presence of relatively normal cholesterol levels. The atherogenic lipid pattern with a relatively normal total cholesterol, with a low HDL, a high LDL/HDL ratio, and hypertriglyceridaemia, should also be excluded. Patients undergoing investigation for coronary heart disease or other vascular disease should have a full lipid profile performed, irrespective of the initial cholesterol findings. It should be a routine procedure to check the cholesterol levels of all family members of coronary patients.

Diet, exercise and weight control

It is our policy in dealing with coronary patients to prescribe a prudent balanced diet aimed at reducing the calorie intake from fat to less than 35%. The carbohydrate intake should be increased to more than 50%, with emphasis on a moderate intake of coarse, high fibre carbohydrate. Less strict dietary intervention may be imposed on patients over 65 years, because of uncertainty of benefit. More strict saturated fat restriction and cholesterol limitation is indicated in coronary patients with hyperlipidaemia. We should aim at reducing fat intake to less than 30% of calories. This is a level which is not easily achieved in high fat consuming communities but it is nevertheless a desirable aspiration. Alcohol and refined carbohydrate must be restricted in the type 4 hyperlipidaemia.

Patients are advised to adopt an active aerobic exercise programme and to reduce weight, when indicated, as added measures to normalise the

Table 10.1 Lipid lowering drugs

Drugs		Efficacy	Dose	Side effects	Cost	Remarks
1. Bile acid sequestrants	Colestipol Cholestyramine	LDL↓ TGS↑ or→ HDL→	8-24 grms	Bloating Constipation	Expensive	Very safe. Needs well motivated patient.
2. Fibric acid	Gemfibrozil Bezafibrate Fenobrate Ciprofibrate Clofibrate	TGS↓ HDL↑ LDL→	600-1200 mgs	None apart from cholelithiasis and ? increased GIT cancer with Clofibrate.	Moderate	Gemfibrozil (Lopid) has been shown to lower coronary mortality. Clofibrate contraindicated because of adverse trial results. Type IIB, III, IV, V
3. HMG CoA reductase inhibitors	Lovostatin Pravastatin Simvastatin	LDL↓ TGS ↓ HDL↑	10-80 mgs	Few Myositis rarely with fibric acid or nicotinic acid. Liver enzymes activity may rise.	Expensive	Highly effective and easily tolerated for severe Type II hyperlipidaemia.
4. Nicotinic acid (Niacin)		TGS↓ LDL↓ HDL↑	1.5-8 grms	Flushing, flatulence, abdominal discomfort, particularly initially.	Cheap	Very effective but needs very well motivated patient and doctor.
5. Probucol		LDL↓ or→ TGS↓ or→ HDL↓		Prolonged QTc. Side effects not significant.	Moderate	Efficacy in doubt. Antioxygent effect may be important in inhibiting atherogenesis.

lipid profile. The advice and supervision of a dietitian is mandatory to obtain early adherence and longterm compliance, and to ensure proper nutritional balance. In most patients, the prudent diet we advocate can be adopted with minor changes in eating habits and cooking techniques, and without increasing cost. These dietary modifications should be adopted by the patient's family. This ensures better longterm compliance with healthy eating and encourages useful primary preventive habits for family members.

In the more severe hyperlipidaemias, and in the intractable cases which show little or no response to dietary measures, chemotherapy may be required. Guidelines for the use of chemotherapy have been published by the National Cholesterol Education Programme (1989) and by the European Atherosclerosis Society (1988).

Table 10.1 lists the drugs available in most western countries and records their principal indications in relation to cholesterol and triglyceride control. The table includes details of dosage, side-effects and cost. Vigorous chemotherapy will substantially reduce cholesterol levels and restore a near normal lipid profile, even in some heterozygous cases.

Drug therapy should not be prescribed without first giving an adequate trial to dietary intervention, combined with weight control and exercise programmes. Secondary hyperlipidaemia, as in patients with renal, pancreatic and thyroid disease, must also be excluded. Subject to these qualifications, arbitrary cut-off values of LDL cholesterol above which medication should be prescribed have been proposed by the National Cholesterol Education Programme (1989). The European Atherosclerosis Group (1988) have also attempted to give cut-off points.

However, arbitrary figures are too simplistic in that several other factors must influence decision-making as well as the LDL and total cholesterol levels. The use of appropriate medication is particularly justified in younger subjects and in those with a high LDL/HDL ratio, in subjects with low HDL levels, in the presence of other risk factors for coronary heart disease, and in subjects with a family and personal history of vascular disease. It needs to be emphasised that our patients with coronary heart disease should receive particular priority as subjects for medication if a normal lipid profile cannot be achieved by dietary and other non-pharmacological means.

Table 10.2, dealing with total cholesterol levels, provides different criteria of risk according to age and was published by the Cholesterol Consensus Conference (NIH Consensus 1985). Table 10.3 refers to LDL levels and provides useful guidelines about management. LDL levels of 160 mg% (3.9 mmol/L) or greater may indicate the need for medication.

Combined therapy may be useful in that it may be more effective, less costly and have a useful synergistic action. The management of severe

Table 10.2 Risk levels mgs% (mmol/L) for moderate and high total cholesterol*

Age (years)	Moderate risk	High risk
20–29	200 to 219 (5.2–5.7)	220 (5.7)
30–39	220 to 239 (5.7–6.2)	240 (6.2)
40	240 to 259 (6.2–6.7)	260 (6.7)

*Consensus Conference on Lipid Lowering. Journal of the American Medical Association 1985; 253:2080

Table 10.3 Cholesterol Consensus Conference* Classification and treatment decisions based on LDL cholesterol in mgm% (mmol/L)

Classification		
130 (3.3)	Desirable LDL cholesterol	
130–159 (3.3–3.6)	Borderline high risk	
160 (3.6)	High risk	
	Initiation level	**Minimal goal**
Dietary treatment		
Without CHD or **two** other risk factors	160 (3.6)	160
With CHD or **two** other risk factors	130 (3.3)	130
Drug treatment:		
Without CHD or **two** other risk factors	190 (3.9)	160
With CHD or **two** other risk factors	160 (3.6)	130

LDL = Low density lipoprotein; CHD = Coronary heart disease
Patients have a lower initiation level and goal if they are at high risk because they already have definite CHD, or because they have any two of the following risk factors: male sex, family history of premature CHD, cigarette smoking, hypertension, low high density lipoprotein, diabetes mellitus, definite cardiovascular or peripheral vascular disease, or severe obesity.
*Source: Archives of Internal Medicine 1988; 148:36-39

hyperlipidaemia may require the advice of a lipidologist or a cardiologist specialising in this area.

There is now evidence that chemotherapy, combined with dietary control, may lead to regression of atherosclerosis in the coronary arteries, and may protect saphenous grafts from atherosclerotic change (Arntzenius et al 1985, Blankenhorn et al 1978, 1987, 1988, Brensike et al 1984, Duffield et al 1983, Nash et al 1984, Nikkila et al 1984). Difficulties encountered in treatment with longterm chemotherapy include cost and side effects. These difficulties are relevant to the successful use of these drugs but the well controlled and well informed patient can usually be motivated to accept such treatment. The advent of the newer drugs, including the HMG

Coenzyme. A reductase inhibitors and the newer fibric acid derivatives, have greatly reduced side effects and have contributed to greater therapeutic efficacy.

REFERENCES

Arntzenius A C, Kromhout D, Borth J D et al 1985 Diet, lipoproteins and the progression of coronary atherosclerosis. The Leiden Intervention Trial. New England Journal of Medicine 312:805-811

Ball K P, Hanington E, McAllen P M et al 1965 Low-fat diet in myocardial infarction. Lancet 2:501-504

Bierenbaum M L, Fleischman A I, Green D P et al 1970 The five year experience of modified fat diets on younger men with coronary heart disease. Circulation 42:943-952

Blankenhorn D H, Brooks S H, Selzer R H, Barndt R Jr 1978 The rate of atherosclerosis change during treatment of hyperlipoproteinaemia. Circulation 57:355-361

Blankenhorn D H, Nessim S A, Johnson R L, Sanmario M E, Azen S P, Cashin-Hemphill L 1987 Beneficial effects of combined colestipol-niacin therapy on coronary atherosclerosis and coronary venous bypass grafts. Journal of the American Medical Association 257:3233-3240

Blankenhorn D H, Johnson R L, El Zein H A, Vailas L I 1988 Dietary fat influences human coronary lesion formation. Circulation 78:89-96

Brensike J F, Levy R I, Kelsey S F et al 1984 Effects on therapy with cholestyramine on progression of coronary atherosclerosis: results of the NHLBI Type 11 Coronary Intervention Study. Circulation 69:313-324

Campeau L, Enjalbert M, Lesperance J et al 1984 The relation of risk factors to the development of atherosclerosis in saphenous-vein bypass grafts and the progression of disease in the native circulation. A study 10 years after aortocoronary bypass surgery. New England Journal of Medicine 311:1329-1332

Canner P L, Berge K G, Wenger N K et al 1986 Fifteen year mortality in Coronary Drug Project patients: long-term benefit with niacin. Journal of the American College of Cardiology 8:1245-1255

Carlson L A, Rosenhammer G 1988 Reduction in mortality in the Stockholm Ischemic Heart Study by combined treatment with clofibrate and nicotinic acid. Acta Medica Scandinavica 223:405-418

Duffield R G, Lewis B, Miller N E, Jamieson C W, Brunt J N, Colchester A C 1983 Treatment of hyperlipidaemia retards progression of symptomatic femoral atherosclerosis. A randomized controlled trail. Lancet 2:639-642

European Atherosclerosis Society 1988 The recognition and management of hyperlipidaemia in adults: a policy statement of the European Atherosclerosis Society. European Heart Journal 9:571-600

Hansen P F, Geill T, Lund E 1962 Dietary fats and thrombosis. Lancet 2:1193-1194

Kallio V, Hamalainen H, Hokkila J, Luurila O J 1979 Reduction in sudden deaths by a multifactorial invervention programme after acute myocardial infarction. Lancet 2:1091-1094

Leren P 1970 The Oslo diet-heart study. Eleven-year report. Circulation 42:935-942

Medical Research Council 1968 Controlled trial of soya-bean oil in myocardial infarction. Lancet 2:693-699

Morrison LM 1960 Diet in coronary atherosclerosis. Journal of the American Medical Association 173:884-888

Mulcahy R, Hickey, N, Maurer, B 1967 Coronary heart disease in women. Study of risk factors in 100 patients less than 60 years of age. Circulation 36:577-586.

Mulcahy R, Hickey N, Maurer B 1967 Coronary heart disease. A study of risk factors in 400 patients under 60 years. Geriatrics 24:106-1014

Nash D T, Gensini G, Esente P 1984 The progression of coronary atherosclerosis. Journal of Cardiac Rehabilitation 4:212-216

National Cholesterol Education Programme 1989 Report of the expert panel on detection, evaluation and treatment of high blood cholesterol in adults. USDHHS, NIH Publication No.89-2925 Bethesda

NIH Consensus Development Conference statement 1985 Lowering blood cholesterol to prevent heart disease. Arteriosclerosis 5:404-412

Nikkila E A, Viikinkoski P, Valle M, Frick M H 1984 Prevention of progression of coronary atherosclerosis by treatment of hyperlipidaemia: a seven year prospective angiographic study. British Medical Journal 289:220-223

Phillips A N, Shaper A G, Pocock S J, Walker M, MacFarlane P W 1988 The role of risk factors in heart attack occurring in men with pre-existing ischaemic heart disease. British Heart Journal 60:404-410

Rose G A, Thomsom W B, Williams R T 1965 Corn oil in treatment of ischaemic heart disease. British Medical Journal 1965 24:1159-1191

Wissler R W, Vesselinovitch D 1983 Combined effects of cholestyramine and probucol on regression of atherosclerosis in rhesus monkey aortas. Applied Pathology 1:89-96

FURTHER READING

Ball M, Mann J (eds) 1988 Lipids and Heart Disease: A Practical Approach, Oxford University Press pp 1-174

Bilheimer D W 1988 Therapeutic control of hyperlipidaemia in the prevention of coronary atherosclerosis: a review of results from recent clinical trials. American Journal of Cardiology 62:J1-9

Billingsworth D R, Bacon S 1989 Treatment of heterozygote familial hypercholesterolaemia with lipid lowering drugs. Arteriosclerosis (suppl 1):1-121

Department of Health & Human Services 1988 The Surgeon General's Report on nutrition and health. US Government printing office, Washington DC USDHHS publication 88-50210

Grundy S M, Bearn A G (eds) 1989 The Role of Cholesterol in Atherosclerosis: New Therapeutic Opportunities. Hanley-Belfus St Louis pp 1-271

National Cholesterol Education Programme 1989 Report of the Expert Panel on Detection, Evaluation and Treatment of High Blood Cholesterol in Adults. USDHHS, NIH Publication No. 89-2925 Bethesda

Witztum J L 1989 Current approaches to drug therapy for the hypercholesterolemic patient. Circulation 80:1101-1114.

11. Obesity

It is customary to measure weight by estimating the subject's Body Mass Index (BMI). A BMI between 20-25 is considered to be normal, less than 20 indicates underweight, above 25 and less than 30 overweight, and 30 or over is defined as obesity. A nomogram is useful to identify the BMI (see Fig. 11.1). There is little evidence that obesity is a primary risk factor for coronary disease, nor is there any evidence that weight change affects the outlook in post-infarction or surgical patients. However, excess weight does

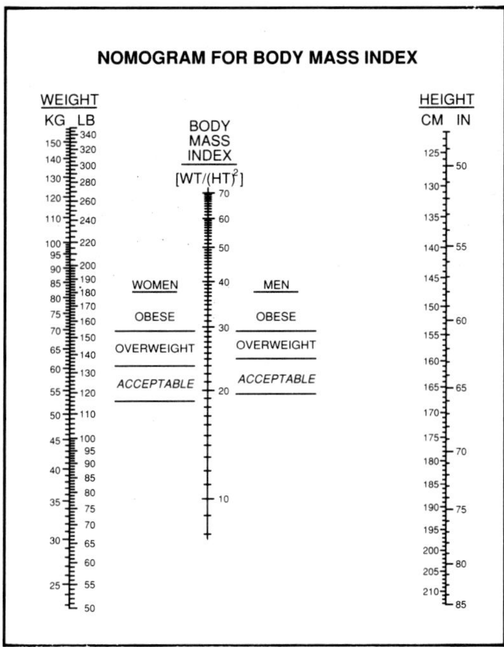

Fig. 11.1 A nomogram for determining body mass index. To determine body mass index, place a straight edge between the body weight on the left-hand column and the height on the right-hand column. The body mass index is at the point where this straight edge connecting height and weight crosses the body mass index line in the middle. (Copyright G A Bray, 1978, reproduced with permission.)

aggravate angina of effort, may contribute to the development of post-myocardial infarction angina, and is a non-specific risk factor for many medical and behavioural problems which are relevant to the management of patients with coronary heart disease. It is an accepted part of rehabilitation and secondary prevention that excessive weight, particularly in those deemed to be obese, should be discouraged, and that compliance with weight reduction may help to assist other life-style changes which may be recommended.

While initial weight reduction after a myocardial infarction has been relatively good in our experience, compliance with weight reduction over the long term in obese patients can be disappointing. We have found obesity to be one of the most intractable conditions to overcome. We did achieve a satisfactory reduction in 33% of our overweight or obese patients (Reid & Mulcahy, 1987), but this was largely achieved in those who were least overweight.

Weight reduction

Success will only be achieved by expert counselling and longterm encouragement and supervision. The advice of a dietitian is essential. It is futile to prescribe a weight-reducing regime without exploring the patient's history in an attempt to define the cause of overweight and the basis of the patient's excessive calorie intake. Identification of the causative background will help considerably in estimating the likelihood of a satisfactory response. For instance, if the patient has been obese since childhood, if overeating is a response to domestic or other intractable stress, or if dietary control leads to depression, the outlook is generally not good. If the weight gain has been of recent origin or is a response to an unusual life event, such as marriage, stopping smoking or a surgical operation, the outlook may be much better. The patient's psychological make-up, particularly in relation to body image, self-esteem and motivation, and his or her response to stress in terms of anxiety and depression, will also determine the likely longterm response to dietary control.

The subject needs to be examined to exclude hyperlipidaemia, Cushings Syndrome and diabetes, and to note the fat distribution. The android type of obesity, where the fat is mostly found in the abdominal region, is easier to treat than the fat of a gynaecoid type, which is found predominantly around the hips and thighs.

Crash dieting should be avoided, not only because it is less likely to succeed in the long run, but also because of possible undesirable physiological effects, such as loss of protein as well as fat. Learning to eat more slowly and keeping a food diary may help. The dietary programme should be carefully planned with longterm aims and objectives clearly defined. Nutritional balance should be assured and deviations from defined dietary guidelines should be avoided. There may be a limited place for anorexogenic drugs to encourage early co-operation but in our experience recourse to such treatment does not augur well for compliance with dietary control. Psychotropic drugs may be rarely helpful and psychotherapy may have a place in compulsive eaters and in those with emotional problems.

Family support and encouragement is essential, as is longterm counselling and supervision. Active aerobic exercise makes a contribution to satisfactory weight reduction but, again, motivation to comply with a programme of adequate duration and intensity is too frequently lacking. The exercise must be graduated in nature and, if it is to play a part in sustained weight control, it needs to be of adequate intensity, not only to increase calorie consumption but also to have an appreciable appetite-suppressing effect and to sublimate any associated stresses which may be contributing to the subject's food dependency.

Excessive and regular alcohol intake is a common cause of obesity in males. In these subjects, alcohol limitation or prohibition is mandatory to achieve satisfactory weight control and to motivate the patient to adopt other life-style changes, such as smoking cessation and adoption of exercise programmes. Repeated measurement of weight, exercise capacity, cholesterol and blood pressure levels may confirm progress and will add an incentive to the subject's compliance.

DIABETES MELLITUS

Diabetes mellitus is frequently alluded to as a risk factor for coronary heart disease. While a high percentage of diabetics are found among coronary patients and while diabetics appear to be particularly prone to coronary heart disease and other vascular complications, there is no incontrovertible evidence that the association is a causative one. There may be confounding factors to account for the association, such as the high fat diet previously prescribed for diabetic patients, a policy which has now been discarded by diabetologists. Hypertriglyceridaemia is also common and may play an adverse role in atherogenesis. Diabetics may be less prone to coronary heart disease in populations with a low fat intake and with low serum cholesterol levels, such as exists in Japan (Marmot et al 1975). There is still some controversy and not a little uncertainty about diabetes as an independent risk factor for coronary disease, nor is there any evidence that good control of diabetes will reduce the patient's propensity to a further coronary attack. The type of vascular disease found to be common and unique in diabetes is a micro-angiopathy not related to classical atherosclerosis (McMillan 1986).

Having said this, it remains that diabetics have a less satisfactory prognosis during the acute stage of myocardial infarction. The sugar levels may be difficult to control at this juncture, as in any acute illness or injury. Control during the acute stage will require careful monitoring of sugar levels and of ketone bodies, with the use of frequent and variable doses of insulin. After recovery, diabetics should aim at optimum control and there should be the same emphasis on the need for risk factor modification in relation to hypertension, obesity, and smoking. Regular aerobic exercise should be recommended, and the traditional high fat diet should be assiduously avoided.

REFERENCES

Marmot M G, Syme S L, Kagan A, Kato H, Cohen J B, Belsky J 1975 Epidemiologic studies of coronary heart disease and stroke in Japanese men living in Japan, Hawaii and California: prevalence of coronary and hypertensive heart disease and associated risk factors. American Journal of Epidemiology 102:514-525

McMillan D E 1986 Monitoring the appearance and progress of blood and vascular abnormalities. In: Davidson JK (ed) Clinical diabetes mellitus, a problem-orientated approach. Thieme, New York, pp 317-28

Reid V, Mulcahy R 1987 Nutrient intakes and dietary compliance in cardiac patients: 6-year follow-up. Human Nutrition Applied Nutrition 41:311-318

12. Hypertension

There is a higher prevalence of hypertension in patients with coronary disease than in the normal population. Hypertension is recognised as one of the three primary risk factors in populations with high mean cholesterol levels. Poorly controlled hypertension is also a risk factor for thrombo-atherosclerotic stroke, peripheral vascular disease and aneurysm, and is significantly associated with haemorrhagic stroke, subarachnoid haemorrhage, left ventricular failure, renal failure and ruptured aneurysm.

Mortality attributed to hypertension has been falling for 50 years or more, so that haemorrhagic stroke, and cardiac and renal failure of hypertensive origin, have become relatively rare causes of death in most western countries today. This can be partly attributed to the gradual progress made in the identification and treatment of hypertension during the past 25-40 years. It may also be attributed to a dramatic decline in the incidence of hypertension secondary to renal disease and other causes, and to their better treatment.

However, the decline in hypertension mortality commenced before the advent of effective treatment of hypertension and before its widespread identification. The earlier mortality decline cannot be fully explained but may be related to the gradual decline of the prevalence of renal disease, and to the substitution by deep freezing and other methods for salt as a food preservative. Despite great difficulties in interpreting the evidence linking salt and hypertension, epidemiological studies leave us in no doubt that populations with high salt intakes have a higher prevalence of hypertension and hypertensive disease. Hypertension is rare in populations with a low salt intake.

Preventive trials of hypertensive treatment leave little doubt that control is successful in reducing the risk of stroke, left ventricular failure and renal failure. However, no such benefit has been reported in these trials in terms of preventing coronary heart disease. This has left us in some doubt about the efficacy of hypertensive control in coronary heart disease prevention, but there is some evidence that a possible beneficial effect of hypertension control in reducing the risk of coronary heart disease may be counterbalanced by the adverse effect which certain hypotensive medications may have on the lipid profile (Ames 1987, Stamler & Stamler 1984). It has been shown that thiazide diuretics and beta-blockers, the most commonly used drugs in the management of hypertension, have an adverse effect through reduction of high density lipoprotein cholesterol and increase in triglyceride levels in the case of selective and non-selective beta-blockers, and similar changes in the case of thiazide diuretics. Beta-blockers with ISA appear to cause little change in the lipid profile (MacMahon et al 1986). These lipid changes are undesirable, particularly in high risk, coronary-prone patients or in those with established disease.

Hypertension and prognosis

Hypertensive patients have a worse prognosis after myocardial infarction than normotensive patients (Graham et al 1978). There are a very few trials reported of the influence of hypertension control in the secondary prevention of coronary heart disease. In a limited non-randomised trial we reported, we found a significant reduction in mortality in hypertensive survivors of a first myocardial infarction who were deemed to be adequately treated during longterm follow up, compared to a group who were inadequately treated or who were poor compliers (Graham et al 1978). The Mayo group, reporting a randomised secondary preventive trial reported beneficial results in their treated group (Connolly et al 1983). It is unlikely that a well designed acceptable trial will ever be conducted in this area for ethical reasons, because of the compelling evidence from primary preventive trials that hypertension benefits from drug and appropriate non-pharmacological treatment, at least in terms of morbidity and mortality from stroke, aneurysm, left ventricular and renal failure. For this reason, and because no deleterious effect of adequate hypertension control has been shown to result in patients with coronary heart disease, the usual principles of management should be applied to the coronary patient.

The following aspects of management need stressing:

* There should be a strong emphasis on non-pharmacological methods, including weight control, calorie and salt limitation, adopting active exercise programmes, and counselling about avoiding and coping with abnormal stress situations. Non-pharmacological measures include control of cigarette smoking, alcohol limitation and control of hyperlipidaemia.

* Hypertensive drugs which adversely affect the lipid profile should be avoided. If possible, thiazide diuretics should not be used in coronary patients, and beta-blockers are also undesirable, although they are

advocated by some physicians because of their reported effect in improving survival after myocardial infarction. Both groups of drugs have been shown to raise LDL and lower HDL cholesterol levels. More research is required to elucidate the exact longterm effect of these and other drugs on the lipid profile. In the meantime it is best to use drugs which do not affect the lipid profile or, preferably, which improve the profile by raising the HDL and lowering the LDL fractions. Of particular interest in this context are the $alpha_1$ adrenergic agents, such as prazosin and doxazin, and the ACE inhibitors.

Thiazides may also adversely affect glucose tolerance and serum potassium levels, and may precipitate gout in susceptible subjects.

* The patient or, exceptionally, a spouse or family member, should be trained to monitor blood pressure. Self-monitoring of blood pressure has proved acceptable to most of our hypertensive patients and plays an important part in improving patient motivation and subsequent compliance with treatment. Patients can be trained to titrate drug dosage and drug regimes, and some become skilled at keeping blood pressure levels at normal or near normal levels. In many, gradual reduction or cessation of drug treatment can be achieved for prolonged periods, particularly if non-pharmacological measures of blood pressure control are adhered to. Quite often, the physician may be unsure of the post-myocardial infarction patient's blood pressure status, because of labile blood pressure levels which may return to normal or near normal at times. In these cases we recommend the routine adoption of non-pharmacological methods of control, and regular self-monitoring of blood pressure levels. Most patients settle at acceptable levels of blood pressure on non-pharmacological treatment, but some will require interrupted or continuous medication.
* Hypertensive patients may become normotensive or even hypotensive after a myocardial infarction. Drug treatment can be suspended in this event but, except in patients with severe left ventricular damage, the blood pressure may return to high pre-infarct levels some weeks or months after the initial event. Non-pharmacological methods of treatment should be routinely advocated in these patients but regular blood pressure checks will be required during follow-up in case drug treatment needs to be resumed.

REFERENCES

Ames R P 1987 The influence of non-beta-blocking drugs on lipid profile; are diuretics outclassed as initial therapy for hypertension? American Heart Journal 114:998-1006

Connolly D C, Elveback L R, Oxman H A 1983 Coronary heart disease in residents of Rochester, Minnesota, 1950-1975 111. Effect of hypertension and its treatment on survival of patients with coronary artery disease. Mayo Clinic Proceedings 58:259-264

Graham I M, Mulcahy R, Hickey N, Daly L 1978 Effect of hypertension and its treatment on progress after myocardial infarction. In: Hjalmarson H, Wilhelmsen L (eds) Acute and long-term medical management of myocardial infarction. Lindgren Molndal, pp 279-284

MacMahon S W, Cutler J A, Furberg C D, Poyne G H 1986 The effects of drug treatment for hypertension on morbidity and mortality from cardiovascular disease: a review of randomized controlled trials. Progress in Cardiovascular Diseases 29:199-218

Mulcahy R, Hickey N, Maurer B 1967 Coronary heart disease in women. Study of risk factors in 100 patients less than 60 years of age. Circulation 36:577-586

Mulcahy R, Hickey N, Maurer B 1969 Coronary heart disease. A study of risk factors in 400 patients under 60 years. Geriatrics 24:106-114

Stamler J, Stamler R 1984 Intervention for the prevention and control of hypertension and atherosclerotic diseases: United States and international experience. American Journal of Medicine 76:13-36

FURTHER READING

Hickey N, Graham I M 1988 Hypertension. Series in Clinical Epidemiology (ed Bourke G) Croom Helm, London

Joint National Committee 1988 Detection, Evaluation and Treatment of High Blood Pressure. Report of the Joint National Committee on Detection, Evaluation and Treatment of High Blood Pressure. USDHHS, NIH Publication No. 88-1088 Bethesda

13. Cigarette smoking

Cigarette smoking has been identified, with hyperlipidaemia and hypertension, as one of the three independent coronary risk factors. It plays an important causative role, particularly in populations with high mean cholesterol levels. Its action in relation to atherosclerosis and the genesis of clinical vascular disease is a complex one, including both atherogenic and thrombogenic mechanisms, and, in the case of coronary heart disease, arrhythmogenic influences. Smoking, because of the numerous and complex substances contained in the inhaled smoke, some of which are toxic, causes multi-system disease over and above its effects on the cardiovascular system.

Epidemiological evidence of the relationship between cigarette smoking and coronary heart disease comes from a variety of prospective and case history studies. Conclusions reached through these studies are congruent with pathological, basic research and animal studies, and with the finding

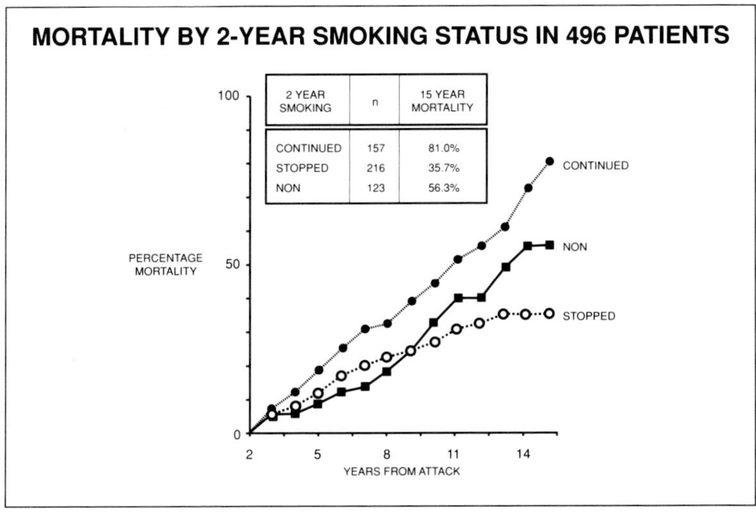

Fig. 13.1. The influence of subsequent cigarette smoking on longterm mortality in males less than 60 years with a first myocardial infarction.

of a reduced incidence of coronary heart disease mortality in primary and secondary prevention studies. The evidence implicating cigarette smoking as an important risk factor for coronary heart disease is incontrovertible and, from the point of view of rehabilitation and secondary prevention, there is now strong evidence that stopping smoking after myocardial infarction reduces the incidence of post-myocardial infarction angina, at least for some years, and favourably affects subsequent recurrence of coronary events, including non-fatal and fatal myocardial infarction, and sudden death (Mulcahy 1983).

Figure 13.1, taken from the British Medical Journal, records our experience of 498 survivors of a first myocardial infarction who had been smokers at the time of the attack. The average annual mortality over 15 years in those who continued afterwards was 10.2% while it was only 3.7% in those who stopped. The initial non-smokers had an intermediate prognosis, principally because they had a higher initial incidence of hypertension and hyperlipidaemia.

Cigar and pipe smoking

We have less certain evidence of the effects of cigar and pipe smoking on coronary heart disease incidence and mortality. Primary cigar and pipe smokers tend not to inhale and may therefore be less vulnerable to vascular damage. However, there are many reports of inhalation among pipe and cigar smokers (and of raised carboxyhaemoglobin levels in such patients) who have changed from cigarette smoking to other forms of tobacco. Once the cigarette smoker has learnt to inhale, he may continue to do so after changing to other forms of tobacco. We have found high carboxyhaemoglobin levels in ex-cigarette smokers who have changed to pipe or cigar smoking (Ronan et al 1981) as have other workers, and, in a follow-up study of 638 patients, we have noted a subsequent mortality in cigar smokers equal to that of patients who continue to smoke cigarettes (Hickey et al 1983). The relationship between cigar and pipe smoking and vascular disease is far less clear than that between cigarette smoking and vascular disease, because of the fewer number of cigar and pipe smokers available for population studies. It is best, in view of this limited information, to recommend that all patients with established vascular disease, including coronary heart disease, should eschew the tobacco habit. No other action taken by us in the secondary prevention of coronary heart disease can equal the benefit in terms of morbidity and mortality of having patients quit the habit.

Factors affecting smoking cessation

Patients who stop abruptly in response to advice are less likely to resume than patients who initially respond by reducing their consumption, with the ultimate intention of stopping (Mulcahy 1984). The less educated are also more difficult to influence and require more sustained counselling and encouragement. The less motivated and those with diminished self-esteem and poor body image, as defined by psychological testing, are also less successful, as is the occasional patient who tends to deny the implications or significance of the heart event. Patients who receive adequate spouse, family, and social or 'buddy' support are more likely to stop. Support must, of course, be based on encouragement, understanding and sympathy. An approach based on moralising, criticism, disapproval or impatience is invariably counterproductive, especially coming from the spouse. Children, if mixing disapproval with expressions of love and concern, can be particularly effective. In our experience, length of time smoking and the quantity smoked do not appear to affect success in cessation.

Stopping smoking

Counselling must first be aimed at establishing the subject's attitude to the smoking habit. It must be established that the subject is anxious to stop. Without this motive, counselling is virtually useless. The great majority of anginal patients, and of survivors of myocardial infarction and coronary artery surgery, are anxious to stop, particularly as they perceive their illness as a life-threatening event. Success in the well motivated patient largely depends on providing accurate, consistent and comprehensive information about the deleterious health effects of smoking and about the many benefits, medical, psychological, social and financial, of stopping. The counsellor must be well informed about these aspects and must have a good knowledge of the scientific basis of the health consequences of the smoking habit. Full information, with reinforcement, based on an understanding and sympathetic approach, will frequently succeed particularly in the early stages when the patient is still conscious of the recent life-threatening event. Counselling can be reinforced by the provision of appropriate literature but we must ensure that the literature is comprehensible to the patient. Our own experience confirms that many of the less educated derive little or no value from health literature, which is written by educated middle class people and can be understood only by their peers (Conroy & Mulcahy 1985).

In counselling about smoking, we must also be careful to advise patients about anticipated side-effects of withdrawal. Withdrawal effects can vary in number and severity, and also in duration. Their severity and duration largely depend on the patient's motivation. The highly motivated patient is frequently surprised by the paucity and mildness of side effects—'it was no problem, doctor, I should have done it long ago!'—while the motivation and commitment of the patient with severe withdrawal effects is always suspect. This relation between motivation and severity of side effects is understandable because the evidence points to withdrawal effects being of psychological rather than physical origin. The fact that the urge to smoke is largely situational confirms this point, as does the very immediate relief of withdrawal effects as soon as the first pull of the cigarette is taken. These facts need to be explained to patients, and particularly to the more recalcitrant ones we encounter.

Side effects, such as depression, irritability and other mood changes, insomnia, feelings of boredom and fatigue, and weight gain should be identified and treated. Regular aerobic exercise is a good antidote to mood change. Advice from a dietitian will frequently prevent weight gain. A sedative at night, or rarely during the day, may be of temporary value in counteracting insomnia and complaints of boredom or tension. Patients should avoid situations and locations associated with smoking, particularly at the early stages. It is implicit in all counselling about withdrawal effects that they are of a temporary nature and that they tend to diminish or resolve with time, with occasional recurrence in certain easily anticipated situations. We can further encourage the subject by emphasising the advantages of becoming a non-smoker, the advantages in terms of health and physical fitness, the social and financial advantages, and, above all, the psychological boost derived from overcoming a strongly addictive habit and of becoming one's own master.

Recidivism

Recidivism is a major problem for the cigarette smoker. Unfortunately, rehabilitation services are seldom of sufficient duration to ensure longterm cessation of smoking, except in the very well motivated. We have followed all our male patients aged less than 60 years with a first myocardial infarction since 1961 and we have paid particular attention to their response to smoking advice and to their longterm smoking habits. Table 13.1 shows the three year cessation rate in our patients over the period 1961-1980 (Hickey et al 1981). The increasing cessation rate over this period of time can be attributed to the improving skill and commitment of our cardiac rehabilitation staff on the one hand, and to the increasing acceptance by the profession and the public of the health hazards of smoking on the other. None of our patients smoked while in the coronary care unit nor did they smoke in the convalescent wards; 86% were still off smoking at the first outpatient visit three weeks after discharge, while 66% were still off smoking at the end of two years (Guiry et al 1987).

We have confirmed the veracity of reported smoking habits in a representative sample of our patients (MacMahon et al 1986). We have looked at some characteristics which might differentiate the longterm compliers

Table 13.1 Response to cigarette smoking advice during six three-year periods from 1961 to 1980. Males under 60 years, first myocardial infarction*

Time interval	Number of initial cigarette smokers	Stopped smokers during follow-up period
1961–1963	63	29 (46.0%)
1964–1966	99	41 (41.4%)
1967–1969	101	57 (56.4%)
1970–1972	123	80 (65.0%)
1973–1975	129	75 (58.1%)
1978–1980	142	98 (70.0%)
Total	657	380 (58.5%)

*Hickey et al 1981. Irish Journal of Medical Science; 150: 262–264.

from those who return to smoking (Conroy et al 1986, Guiry et al 1987). The less educated and the lower income groups are relatively poor compliers compared to the more educated and the higher occupational groups. Those who return to smoking are also less motivated about early return to work, adopting longterm exercise programmes, and achieving weight control. There is a complex relationship between education, ability to respond to counselling, motivation over the long term, and other personality characteristics which we must be aware of. The poor complier can usually be identified by the experienced clinician and health worker. It does not require elaborate, questionnaires to determine psychological or attitudinal responses, nor are these questionnaires of proven value in relation to the practical results of skilled counselling. We do, however, need to provide special attention to the perceived poor complier. In particular, counselling may need to be repeated over many months to maintain reinforcement. Such repeated counselling can ultimately achieve the success which initially appears to be difficult or impossible.

The prevention of recidivism is a special area where repeated review and encouragement may play a very useful role. Patients must be made aware that, while withdrawal effects tend to subside gradually, they may return acutely in special high risk situations, such as social gatherings and in other convivial circumstances, where group smoking and cigarette offering is commonly the rule. With the resolution of withdrawal effects goes a diminishing recollection of the difficulties experienced in overcoming a highly addictive habit. The ex-smoker tends to forget how difficult it was to stop smoking. This may lead to a sense of complacency about one's dependency on tobacco, so that one can yield to the sudden unexpected return of withdrawal effects by accepting a proferred cigarette. That single cigarette may be the downfall of the victim and will often lead to a return of dependency and to a gradual resumption of the smoking habit. The ex-smoker must be urged never to smoke a cigarette TODAY, and never to smoke the first cigarette.

Success in remaining off smoking, particularly in the early stages after discharge from hospital, will be influenced by the advice we give as part of secondary prevention counselling:

- Avoid situations and locations associated with the smoking habit
- Physical exercise or other leisure pursuits may reduce dependency on smoking
- The spouse and family members should stop smoking or avoid smoking in the patient's presence
- Significant side effects should be discussed and may be alleviated by temporary measures such as a mild tranquilliser
- There are aids to smoking control, such as nicotine chewing gum and transdermal patches, hypnosis, and acupuncture. However, they are simply aids, and their need may be an expression of poor motivation on the patient's part. Their success rate leaves much to be desired
- Aversion techniques have been described in certain intractable cases and have apparently had some success
- Inducement techniques may be helpful, particularly in the group or corporate setting. Inducements may be financial or otherwise. Success here clearly depends on the patient's motivation as well as on the strength of the inducement.

In a minority of cases we fail to get our patients to stop smoking. These patients need understanding and continued support. Impatience or criticism on the part of the doctor, spouse or family is counter-productive. As a second best, we have to reduce the impact of smoking by having the patient smoke fewer cigarettes, reduce inhalation and discard a longer butt. The following advice may be appropriate under these circumstances:

- Smoke a cigarette which has a low tar and nicotine content. The tar and nicotine content of all the well-known cigarettes has been listed and information about them can be obtained from your Heart or Cancer Foundation, or from your Ministry of Health
- Smoke less of each cigarette so that the butt becomes progressively longer
- Gradually reduce the intake of tar and nicotine into your lungs by cutting down on your inhaling. Avoid inhaling every second puff at the beginning and gradually decrease the frequency and depth of inhalation afterwards
- Set out non-smoking periods for yourself each day
- Set out non-smoking locations for yourself such as the car, your bedroom or in the presence of your children
- Never offer or accept a cigarette.

REFERENCES

Conroy R M, Mulcahy R 1985 Readability of literature written for cardiac patients. Clinical Cardiology 8:104-106

Conroy R, Mulcahy R, Graham I, Reid V, Cahill S 1986 Prediction of patient response to risk factor modification advice after admission for unstable angina or myocardial infarction. Journal of Cardiopulmonary Rehabilitation 6:344-357

Guiry E, Conroy R M, Hickey N, Mulcahy R 1987 Psychological response to an acute coronary event and its effect on subsequent rehabilitation and lifestyle change. Clinical Cardiology 10:256-260

Hickey N, Graham I, Kennedy C, Daly L, Mulcahy R 1981 Trends in response to anti-smoking advice in patients with coronary heart disease between 1961 and 1975. Irish Journal of Medical Science 150:262-264

Hickey N, Mulcahy R, Daly L, Graham I, O'Donoghue S, Kennedy C 1983 Cigar and pipe smoking related to four year survival of coronary patients. British Heart Journal 49:423-426

MacMahon S W, Cutler J A, Furberg C D, Poyne G H 1986 The effects of drug treatment for hypertension on morbidity and mortality from cardiovascular disease: a review of randomised controlled trials. Progress in Cardiovascular Disease 29:199-218

Mulcahy R 1983 Influence of cigarette smoking on morbidity and mortality after myocardial infarction. British Heart Journal 49:410-415

Mulcahy R 1984 Cessation of smoking. Proceedings of the International Symposium on Cardiac Rehabilitation and Secondary Prevention (abstract). Munich

Ronan G, Graham I M, Hickey N, Mulcahy R 1981 The reliability of smoking history amongst survivors of myocardial infarction. British Journal of Addiction 76:425-428

FURTHER READING

NIH Publication No. 86-2178 1986 Clinical opportunities for smoking intervention—a guide for the busy physician. USDHHS, Bethesda

NIH Publication No. 89-8411 1989 Reducing the health consequences of smoking: 25 years of progress. A report of the Surgeon General. USDHHS, Bethesda

PSH Publication No. 1103 1964 Smoking and health. Report of the advisory committee to the Surgeon General of the public health. USDHEW, Bethesda

14. Exercise

Cardiac rehabilitation is inseparable from exercise programmes and the encouragement of exercise training as an integral part of returning to a normal good quality life. Indeed, the exercise component of rehabilitation can sometimes be the core of the entire programme and may dominate or replace other equally important aspects of management.

Is lack of exercise an independent risk factor?

There is still no agreement about the role of exercise as an independent factor in the prevention of coronary heart disease. Many studies of the healthy population confirm that those who are physically active have a lower incidence and mortality from coronary heart disease. However, there are a number of confounding variables which may influence a propensity to coronary heart disease and which may be difficult to separate from the exercise habit. Because of these conflicting factors, it is difficult to assess the exact aetiological role of exercise. Active people tend to be lighter, to smoke less, to be more health conscious in terms of diet, smoking and alcohol abuse, and to have healthier lipid profiles and lower blood pressure (Hickey et al 1975). In addition, preselection is another confounding factor, where healthy people are more likely to become active and to indulge in sport than unhealthy people.

The same difficulties exist in interpreting the role of exercise in patients with coronary heart disease. Again, many studies show a marginal or non-significant advantage in those who adopt active exercise and who show an appropriate training effect, but conclusions about the independent contribution of exercise cannot be resolved because of other confounding behavioural and prognostic factors. A recent meta-analysis of 14 individual randomised trials of exercise in secondary prevention programmes confirms that active subjects after infarction enjoy a 25% better prognosis than those who are inactive (Oldridge et al 1988). The authors maintain that this advantage can be attributed to a partial independent influence of training.

Johansson and colleagues from Sweden (Johansson et al 1988), in a study of 7495 healthy males, and a secondary prevention study of 1273 male survivors of a first myocardial infarction, concluded that the better outlook in active people could be attributed entirely to their more favourable risk factor profiles.

THE BENEFITS OF EXERCISE

Leaving aside the question of exercise as an independent factor in reducing further coronary events, there are a number of clearly established advantages to be gained by appropriate physical activity programmes to justify their routine adoption in patients following myocardial infarction, coronary artery surgery and in those with angina of effort. Regular exercise contributes to musculoskeletal and cardiovascular fitness, and to improved peripheral utilisation of oxygen. These effects become manifest in many patients with angina of effort, with or without previous myocardial infarction. Graduated aerobic exercise, combined where necessary with the use of medication to raise the pain threshold, and with risk factor modification, leads, in our experience, to considerable amelioration and, not infrequently, resolution of anginal pain. This result can be achieved within some weeks or months. The beneficial effect of exercise in the management of chronic angina of effort has been reported elsewhere (Redwood et al 1972, Kennedy et al 1976). Benefit may be attributed to more efficient oxygen utilisation by the cardiac and peripheral muscles, and possibly to improved collateral circulation and capillarisation of the ischaemic heart muscle.

Exercise training has useful metabolic effects in terms of reducing triglycerides and in increasing HDL cholesterol levels, in improving sugar metabolism and in maintaining lower blood pressure levels and lower weight. Regular physical exercise improves quality of life through a greater feeling of well-being and a reduced tendency to depression, anxiety and chronic tension, and to a modification of type A behaviour. Self-esteem and motivation tend to improve in active people and may contribute to better compliance with smoking and weight control, and dietary change. The widespread attention to exercise programmes among rehabilitation groups testifies to the importance attached to these programmes as an integral part of cardiac rehabilitation.

Designing exercise programmes

The indication for exercise testing, the techniques and the standard protocols used, and the measurement of exercise capacity and of changes in exercise capacity, are fully reviewed elsewhere (Ekelund et al 1988). Improvement in exercise capacity and in training can be determined by simple clinical means such as measuring resting pulse rate, and achieving a slower pulse rate in response to a fixed amount of exercise.

Certain principles should be adopted in designing an exercise programme for patients recovering from a myocardial infarction or coronary artery surgery. The programme should be safe and acceptable to the patient in terms of feasibility. Thus, it must suit the patient's inclinations, circumstances and preferences. Exercise which is enjoyable or useful, or both, should be prescribed if longterm compliance is to be achieved. There is little point in starting an exercise programme and achieving a satisfactory training effect if one resumes sedentary habits after the early stages of recovery. Exercise should be aerobic in nature—that is, it should involve increased oxygen consumption with large muscle activity and movement. There are some advantages in adding a limited isometric component to increase muscle strength and stamina. The exercise programme should aim at a gradual increase in the training effect by graduated symptom-limited exercise. There is no special virtue in advising an advanced degree of training as the physical and psychological advantages of exercise will be achieved by a moderate training effect, and the dangers of excessively vigorous, sustained or competitive exercise should be avoided.

Exercise and training programmes are safe after myocardial infarction and cardiac surgery subject to the following conditions:

* That there are no marked ischaemic changes or ventricular ectopic rhythms in response to the exercise stress test
* That the intensity of the prescribed exercise is not excessive
* That the patient's heart rate must not rise above 80-85% of the estimated maximum heart rate (Hossack & Hartwig 1982).

Within the stated limits of any exercise programme, whether supervised or not, there appears to be little risk of inducing fresh infarctions or life-threatening arrhythmias (Van Camp & Peterson 1986, Haskell 1978).

To achieve and maintain an appropriate training effect, the exercise process must be adequate in terms of intensity, duration and frequency, and should be practised regularly. The greatest single problem attending rehabilitation programmes is the poor longterm compliance rates and our failure to understand and to remedy the causes of poor compliance. Most rehabilitation exercise programmes are designed to achieve a training effect within a few months of discharge from hospital. But insufficient attention is paid to instructing the patient about the causes and circumstances leading to recidivism. Drop-out is common, and, in the few longterm studies reported, there is a gradual increase in drop-out numbers so that longterm compliance tends to be patchy and disappointing.

Group exercise programmes

Many types of exercise programmes have been devised, particularly in the early convalescent stages after myocardial infarction and coronary artery surgery. Most centres advocate group exercise programmes where a routine of calisthenics and aerobic exercises is conducted and designed according to the exercise capacity and the progress achieved by each subject. The programmes vary in the frequency and duration of sessions, and the duration of the programme. They all share the same advantage in that patients can be under professional surveillance during the earlier stages of recovery and they can receive repeated counselling about home-based exercise and about other desirable life-style and behavioural recommendations. As a general rule, group sessions are held three times each week, and the full programme may last from 8 to 12 weeks. Some patients will make quicker progress than others, and may therefore require a shorter programme. Sessions of about one to one and a half hours are required to allow for a warming up period, an adequate exercise session, a cooling down period, and an opportunity to provide a short counselling session. A programme longer than 12 weeks is seldom necessary as patients will usually have reached their optimum training effect by then. An optimum effect should be 70-80% of maximum capacity as measured by maximum heart rate (maximum heart rate = 220 − age).

Group exercise programmes will allow gradual assessment of progress, including the patient's exercise capacity, and of fitness to return to work and a normal life. Programmes are to be recommended in the early stages of rehabilitation, and should be organised in the hospital or in an appropriate institution within a week or two after the patient's discharge. It is necessary to have staff trained in cardio-respiratory resuscitation present and to have the necessary resuscitation equipment available. Telemetry is often employed during exercise sessions but there is still uncertainty about its value or necessity (American College of Cardiology 1986). Perhaps it should be reserved for high risk cases who are undergoing early exercise training.

Group exercise programmes are not always feasible because of logistic and other difficulties. Facilities may be lacking in some hospitals, the physicians may not be properly motivated, the patients may be unwilling or unable to return to the hospital after discharge, and the number of patients requiring the facility may be too few. In fact, group exercise programmes are not necessary for those survivors of myocardial infarction and coronary surgery who are asymptomatic and deemed to be at low risk. One can substitute home exercise programmes and combine them with visits to a rehabilitation and secondary prevention outpatient clinic (Konig et al 1983, DeBusk et al 1985).

In our programme at St. Vincent's Hospital, now in existence since 1966, we have not employed group exercise programmes (Hickey & Mulcahy 1985). Instead we advise home-based programmes tailored to each patient's perceived exercise capacity. We see each patient at regular intervals of three weeks, three, six, and 12 months after a myocardial infarction, and subsequently at yearly intervals. At each visit the patient's cardiovascular status and reported life-style habits are reviewed, and advice about life-style treatment is reinforced. Our programme has the advantage of providing a longterm follow-up facility, and thus overcomes many problems arising from poor longterm compliance. This follow-up can be provided without any major logistic difficulties. It is a service which can be usefully provided after group exercise programmes.

The principles guiding exercise programmes are routinely applied. Exercise should be adequate in terms of frequency, intensity and duration. It should be aerobic in nature and symptom-limited, and it should be enjoyed by the patient, or at least it should become an integral and useful part of the patient's daily life. Our emphasis, particularly during the early months, is on walking as being the most feasible and physiological form of aerobic exercise available to all patients. We advise patients to adopt graduated walking in terms of duration and intensity, from the time of discharge, and we advocate reaching a daily distance of symptom-limited walking of five kilometres (three miles) by the first outpatient visit. Most patients can achieve this objective but those with impaired left ventricular function, or with other vascular or non-vascular disabilities, may require a more graduated and more delayed approach to achieving a training effect.

In advocating a walking programme, we lay down certain guidelines, including advice about resting after meals, wearing suitable clothing and shoes (in an urban setting, running shoes are best), seeking family support and participation, and choosing pleasant and appropriate surroundings. Patients are taught to recognise chest pain, dyspnoea on exertion and fatigue, and to report these at a subsequent visit. The patient's response to exercise in terms of its intensity and of symptoms produced allows us to evaluate exercise capacity, and we find this is a satisfactory substitute for information about exercise capacity derived from exercise testing.

At a later stage of rehabilitation we review the patient's problems and circumstances, and we may encourage other aerobic activities, such as swimming, cycling, golf, tennis, and jog-walking or jogging. Most of our patients adhere to walking as the mainstay of their exercise programme, but an eclectic interest in exercise is encouraged and some calisthenics or isometric-type exercises are not discouraged, with the exception of vigorous weight-lifting and press-ups. Walking has the advantage in terms of long-term compliance that many subjects will acquire the same commitment to walking that one finds in joggers and runners. The commitment takes some time to develop and therefore early adherence to programmes is vital. Patients can be encouraged to walk part or all of the way to or from work, to walk in salubrious surroundings and at weekends with family members or friends, to join a walking club or to acquire a dog. Whether combined with other aerobic activities or not, symptom-limited walking will achieve a training effect which is adequate in musculoskeletal, cardiorespiratory and metabolic terms, and which contributes to optimum quality of life and pyschological well-being. This training effect is at least equivalent to that achieved after group exercise programmes (De Busk et al 1985).

As reported by other workers (De Busk et al 1985), home-based, symptom-limited walking has been a safe recommendation in our hands. In a follow-up of 390 male patients under 60 years with a first myocardial infarction seen between 1966 and 1975 inclusive, no death was recorded during walking exercise, apart from one patient who died suddenly while training greyhounds. Reported compliance with exercise programmes (21 miles or 36 kilometres walking or more a week) was noted after 3 years in 124 of 244 patients who had been sedentary at the time of the initial attack (Mulcahy 1985).

Exercise testing

Exercise tests are not routinely performed during the follow-up period nor do we measure exercise capacity, apart from assessing the patient's reported exercise experience at each follow-up visit. However, exercise testing can be valuable in selected cases, such as patients with angina of effort who may require further investigation, those who may be symptomatic without obvious cause, and patients who require reassurance or who are lacking in motivation.

It is policy to assess a patient's potential exercise capacity before precribing an early training programme. Capacity mainly depends on left ventricular function and on the presence and severity of post-myocardial infarction angina. Limitations may be caused by other non-cardiac symptoms, such as intermittent claudication, dyspnoea of respiratory origin, fatigue of physical and psychological origins, disability caused by musculoskeletal disease, and gross obesity and other chronic systemic disease. Assessment of exercise capacity is an integral part of risk stratification and depends in the main on assessing left ventricular function, which again depends on evaluating the degree of left ventricular damage. It is now widely advocated that such assessment is best carried out by doing a submaximal exercise ECG before discharge from hospital or within a few weeks of discharge. The evidence favouring routine pre-discharge submaximal exercise testing is far from convincing (Cleempoel et al 1988) and, in my view, testing is not necessary to supplement good clinical evaluation in most patients.

If necessary, and if the circumstances demand it, exercise testing may be supplemented by other methods of evaluating left ventricular function and left ventricular damage. Routine echocardiography to check left ventricular function and dimensions is useful, and adds little to the cost of rehabilitation. Exercise thallium and dipyridamole stress testing, MUGA scan and ventriculography have a place in evaluating left ventricular function but they are not necessary or desirable in the majority of patients before prescribing an exercise programme. Excessive dependence on tests, prominent in some centres today, should be avoided. Their routine use in cardiac rehabilitation is undesirable because of their cost and the logistic problems created by their widespread use, resources which are unlikely to be available to deal with all the cardiac patients who are in need of effective rehabilitation services.

Careful clinical evaluation of left ventricular function, as described on page 51, when combined with the patient's reported exercise tolerance and any limiting symptoms which may be present during the early stages of home-based exercise, is sufficient from the practical point of view to permit us to provide clear longterm guidelines about exercise capabilities. We do not do routine pre-discharge exercise ECGs nor do we do routine exercise tests early in convalescence. However, in patients limited by angina, dyspnoea, unusual fatigue, palpitation or lack of confidence and motivation, special investigations of exercise capacity and left ventricular function can be helpful in planning an exercise prescription, or in deciding about the need for further investigation and treatment.

Exercise and the damaged left ventricle

Patients with extensive heart muscle damage or with other cardiac problems leading to left ventricular impairment are frequently denied the advantages of aerobic exercise. For both medical and psychological reasons, caution must be observed in prescribing exercise for such patients, but a remarkable degree of improvement in exercise capacity can be safely achieved in patients with limited left ventricular function by slow graduated walking and gentle calisthenics (Squires et al 1987, Arvan 1988). Poor left ventricular function spells a higher risk of complications and early death after myocardial infarction, but this higher risk, compared to that of patients with uncomplicated attacks, is most evident in the first year after infarction. It tends to be less so afterwards (Weinblatt et al 1968). Patients with impaired left ventricular function can achieve a useful degree of symptom-free exercise and training with a well modulated exercise prescription, if combined with an adequate initial period of rest during early convalescence and with appropriate inotropic support and risk factor modification. These patients can be monitored by tests of left ventricular function and by Holter monitoring, but a satisfactory exercise tolerance in itself gives reassuring support to continued activity. Improvement is difficult to achieve in patients with severely impaired left ventricular function, where impaired function is associated with active myocardial ischaemia (Arvan 1988).

Age

Age is not a bar to exercise after myocardial infarction and coronary artery surgery. While exercise programmes must obviously be tailored to the older person's capacity and inclinations, the same physical and psychological advantages of regular aerobic activity and its training effect can be expected and will greatly add to the advantages of successful rehabilitation.

Unexpected limitations

Patients should be advised to report any unusual or unexpected limitation in exercise capacity caused by chest pain, dyspnoea, fatigue, palpitation, dizziness or syncope. They should also be cautioned against adopting excessively strenuous, sustained or competitive exercise. A compulsive tendency to increase activity beyond reasonable levels should be discouraged, not only because of the hazards involved but also because there is no added benefit to be derived from more than moderate fitness.

SEXUAL ACTIVITY DURING REHABILITATION

Implicit in a return to a normal and a good quality of life, for some patients at least, is a resumption of normal sexual activity. Sex counselling is one of the most neglected areas in cardiac rehabilitation. Patients will seldom raise questions in this area and most health professionals are reluctant to open a discussion on such a personal matter, perhaps through lack of confidence in dealing with the subject. Libido and sexual performance, at least in the male, are sensitive to psychological influences, and may be seriously impaired in patients who have suffered a life-threatening event, with its concomitant loss of self-esteem, and with possible mood changes of anxiety, depression and insecurity. Sexual function may be further impaired by medications, and particularly by some hypotensive drugs.

There is no reason to believe that sexual activity or intercourse, as normally practised by the patient in conventional circumstances, is likely to precipitate a fresh myocardial infarction or life-threatening arrhythmia, nor is there any evidence that all sexual activity need be suspended for a prolonged period after return home. A restrictive approach need not be adopted. Patients should be advised that diminished sexual interest and activity are a normal and usually temporary response to any significant illness. Patients on drugs, such as beta-blockers or diuretics, which cause partial or complete impotence, should, if desired by themselves or the spouse, be offered the opportunity of altering medication, if a suitable and effective alternative drug or drug regime can be provided.

REFERENCES

American College of Cardiology 1986. Position report on cardiac rehabilitation. Recommendations of the American College of Cardiology. Journal of the American College of Cardiology 7:451-453

Arvan S 1988 Exercise performance of the high risk acute myocardial infarction patient after cardiac rehabilitation. American Journal of Cardiology 62:197-201

Cleempoel H, Vainsel H, Dramaix M et al 1988 Limitations on the prognostic value of predischarge data after myocardial infarction. British Heart Journal 60:98-103

DeBusk R F, Haskell W L, Miller N H et al 1985 Medically directed at-home rehabilitation soon after clinically uncomplicated acute myocardial infarction: a new model for patient care. American Journal of Cardiology 55:251-257

Ekelund L G, Haskell W L, Johnson J L, Whalley F S, Criqui M H, Sheps D S 1988 Physical fitness as a predictor of cardiovascular mortality in asymptomatic North American men. The Lipid Research Clinic's Mortality Follow-up Study. New England Journal of Medicine 319: 1379-1384

Haskell W L 1978 Cardiovascular complications during exercise training for cardiac patients. Circulation 57:920-924

Hickey, N, Mulcahy R, Bourke G, Graham I, Wilson-Davis K 1975 Study of coronary risk factors related to physical activity in 15,171 men. British Medical Journal 10:256-260.

Hickey N, Mulcahy R 1985 Cardiac rehabilitation program: St Vincent's Hospital rehabilitation programme. Journal of Cardiac Rehabilitation 5:386-388

Hossack K F , Hartwig R 1982 Cardiac arrest associated with supervised cardiac rehabilitation. Journal of Cardiac Rehabilitation 2:402-408

Johansson S, Rosengren A, Tsipogianni A, Ulvenstan G, Wiklund I, Wilhelmsen L 1988 Physical inactivity as a risk factor for primary and secondary coronary events in Gotenborg, Sweden. European Heart Journal 9:L8-19

Kennedy C C, Spiekerman R E, Lindsay M I Jr et al 1976 One-year graduated exercise program for men with angina pectoris. Evaluation by physiologic studies and coronary arteriography. Mayo Clinic Proceedings 51:231-236.

Konig K 1983. Home-based informal rehabilitation. In: Konig K, Denolin H, Dorossiev D (eds) Myocardial infarction, how to prevent, how to rehabilitate (2nd edition). Boehringer Mannheim, pp 163-165

Mulcahy R 1985 The virtues of physical activity in secondary prevention of coronary heart disease. Tromso seminar 'The good things of life' (unpublished)

Oldridge N B, Guyatt G H, Fischer M E, Rimm A A 1988 Cardiac rehabilitation after myocardial infarction. Combined experience of randomized clinical trials. Journal of the American Medical Association 260:945-950

Redwood, D R, Rosing D R, Epstein S E 1972 Circulatory and symptomatic effects of physical training in patients with coronary-artery disease and angina pectoris. New England Journal of Medicine 286:959-965

Squires R W, Lavie C J, Brandt T R, Gau F T, Bailey K R 1987 Cardiac rehabilitation in patients with severe ischaemic left ventricular dysfunction. Mayo Clinic Proceedings 62:997-1002

Van Camp S P, Peterson R A 1986 Cardiovascular complications of outpatient cardiac rehabilitation programs. Journal of the American Medical Association 256:1160-1163

Weinblatt E, Shapiro S, Frank C W, Sager R V 1968 Prognosis of men after first myocardial infarction: mortality and first recurrence in relation to select parameters. American Journal of Public Health 58:1329-1347

FURTHER READING

Brochier M L, Julian D G (eds) 1988 Physical training in patients with heart disease: training in coronary disease. 2nd workshop, European Heart Journal 9:M1-46

Dishman R K (ed) 1988 Exercise Adherence, Its Impact on Public Health. Human Kinetics Books, Champaign

Fardy P S, Yanowitz F G, Wilson P A (eds) 1988 Cardiac rehabilitation, adult fitness and exercise testing. 2nd edition. Lea and Febiger, Philadelphia

Fletcher G F (ed) 1988 Exercise in the practice of medicine 2nd edition. Futura, New York

Shephard R J 1989 Exercise in secondary and tertiary rehabilitation: costs and benefits. Journal of Cardiopulmonary Rehabilitation 9:188-194

Wegner N K (ed) 1985 Exercise and the heart. 2nd edition. Cardiovascular Clinics. F A Davis, Philadephia

15. Psychological aspects of rehabilitation

While many patients will make a satisfactory psychological recovery after a heart attack, with little or no counselling or rehabilitation assistance, the management of immediate and delayed psychological reactions is a crucial part of rehabilitation. Psychological well-being is an integral component of a good quality of life. The patient's mood will have an important influence on other aspects of post-infarction behaviour and life-style. Similar psychological problems may present themselves after coronary artery surgery and angioplasty, but surgical patients require specific pre-operative counselling to anticipate and prevent post-operative mood changes. Patients with chronic angina of effort also require psychological assessment as part of the rehabilitation process.

Anxiety and depression

The immediate psychological impact of a heart attack is evoked by its unexpected and sudden onset, and by the patient's perception of the attack as a serious life-threatening event. Although the degree of anxiety is not related to the severity of the attack, mortality looms large in the patients mind, perhaps for the first time, and the security and the structure of the patient's life virtually disintegrates. These perceptions spell anxiety and loss of confidence and self-esteem. Anxiety proves to be the first and the most obtrusive reaction at this early stage. Although the symptoms of anxiety may not be readily apparent to the doctor or nurse, it is usually present in some measure, except perhaps in the occasional patient who has the capacity to deny the significance of the event.

For practical purposes, anxiety and depression will be identified by the clinician or trained nurse. Appropriately designed questionnaires are frequently employed to identify mood changes, but they are instruments for research and in our experience have no practical function for most patients. A simple questionnaire, as illustrated (Table 5.1) may be useful to follow progress, but the use of questionnaires during the acute stage should be confined to certain problem patients. They are best administered by a psychologist.

The better educated are less prone to depression but anxiety is not obviously related to education or gender (Guiry et al 1987). However, there are no hard and fast rules to guide us about the vulnerability to mood changes of the individual patient.

During the early days, as the patient adapts to this unexpected circumstance and as the thought of an early demise recedes, anxiety tends to diminish, only to be replaced by depression as the realities of the illness and its likely effect on the patient's future becomes more manifest. Anxiety may recur from time to time, particularly when the patient is discharged from the security of the coronary care unit or the hospital, but depression tends to be more long-lasting because of the perceived longterm effects of the patient's illness.

Both anxiety and depression are normal reactions under the circumstances but, with proper counselling and management, these mood changes need only be temporary and should not lead to any significant disablement. In the exceptional case, when anxiety, depression or other mood change prove intractable and fail to respond to good management, we can usually anticipate that the patient was prone to such changes prior to the illness. If excessively severe or prolonged, both anxiety and depression will impair the patient's recovery in terms of return to a normal social, professional, sexual and vocational life, and may lead to significant disruption of the patient's relationship with family, friends and employer. In particular, the motivation required to comply with desirable life-style changes and risk factor modification will be impaired, thus adding to the patient's risk of further illness.

The importance of good communication

The essence of our approach to counteracting anxiety and to preventing subsequent depression is early and good communication between the patient and the attending health professionals. It is essential, therefore, that the nurses in coronary care should be trained in the skills of communication, and that the physician, the resident doctors, the dietitian, social worker and the physiotherapist should possess these skills. Early and ample explanation of coronary care procedures will help the patient to understand the purpose of early management. Explanations of the nature, extent and severity of the heart attack should be realistic and comprehensible. We need to emphasise that the critical high risk stage is generally short, and that measures to anticipate, prevent and treat complications during this critical stage are in hand.

At an early stage, too, it is wise to discuss the cause or causes of the heart attack. One factor provoking anxiety is the patient's ignorance of a cause of his or her illness. 'Why should it happen to me?' Another is the perception that, because no cause is apparent, there is a likelihood of recurrence. The risk factor basis of causation should be simply and clearly explained, with an assurance that such factors will be sought and eliminated if possible, thus reducing the risk of further events. The patient's perception that effective steps will be taken to prevent a recurrence or to prevent complications is the key to reducing early anxiety, and subsequently to increasing the patient's confidence and preventing depression.

The key to effective psychotherapy, both in the early stages in coronary care and in the convalescent wards, and subsequently after discharge, rests on well informed, realistic, consistent and easily understood communication with the patient and family members. Spouse and family members must also be included as their own anxiety may be severe and may be transmitted to the patient. Family and social support are crucial in psychosocial recovery.

Uncertainty, based on poor communication, particularly with the physician in charge, and inconsistent opinions and advice from different health professionals, not only fail to cope with anxiety and depression, but may well aggravate these disabling mood changes. Our counselling must be based on a full knowledge of the natural history of the disease, and on the good progress which can be anticipated in most patients who conform to the guidelines we prescribe, and who comply with recommended treatment methods. Counselling should also take into account our ability to stratify patients into different categories of risk. We can usually recommend a return to a completely normal life in every respect and we can often promise a better quality of life if patients will comply with our life-style guidelines. With appropriate counselling, we found that 70% of 150 patients recovering from a first infarction reported having a better quality of life 12 months after the initial event, compared to their pre-illness status (Conroy & Mulcahy 1989, Conroy et al 1989).

In those patients with more severe or disabling heart damage, or who have other vascular or non-vascular disabilities, while acknowledging the need for certain restrictions and the possibility of further complications or events, we can underline the relatively good prognosis in terms of survival and quality of life which can be enjoyed by many in these circumstances. Even in patients with end-stage or near end-stage disease we can provide a measure of comfort and an alleviation of anxiety if our counselling combines a realistic with a concerned approach, and with an assurance that all is being done to maintain life, comfort and freedom from complications.

Because good and well informed communication is the key to the control of anxiety and depression, and because such communication requires considerable clinical knowledge and experience, counselling is best conducted by the physician and nurses, with co-operation from other health professionals. The psychologist and psychiatrist, in my experience, do not have a dominant role to play in rehabilitation services, except in unusual cases when patients' symptoms appear to be intractable or where there are more profound psychological or psychiatric problems which may be of long standing and may have been present before the coronary event. A psychologist, specially trained in dealing with addictive conditions, may be required to deal with intractable compliance problems, particularly in relation to smoking and obesity. Individual counselling is necessary at the early stages of recovery, but psychosocial aspects can be effectively dealt with later, either individually or at group sessions.

The role of drugs

We seldom require to have recourse to tranquillisers or other psychotropic drugs for the alleviation of anxiety, nor do we commonly employ drugs in the management of depression. If patients fail to respond to counselling and explanation, the assistance of a clinical psychologist or psychiatrist should then be sought.

Caution has been advised in the past when prescribing psychotropic drugs to patients with coronary heart disease who may be prone to drug-induced arrhythmias. There is now considerable doubt about the arrhythmogenic dangers of the MAO inhibitors and the phenothiazines when used in therapeutic dosages (Stern 1987). Except perhaps in patients with chronic ventricular arrhythmias, we would accept the use of these drugs in coronary patients based on psychiatric indications.

Denial

Some patients respond to a heart attack, and to many other life emergencies, by denial. This response may be short-lived or may persist. Denial may be beneficial in the sense that it reduces the risk of anxiety, depression and other mood changes, and tends to maintain self-esteem and a sense of security. Denial is perhaps an advantage to patients in these respects but it decreases the likelihood of compliance with necessary treatment procedures and to desirable life-style changes. These patients need particular attention because of their reluctance to accept professional advice which may conflict with their own perceived needs and inclinations. In a few cases, denial may lead to hostility directed at the physician, nursing staff or family. In some cases an advisory role may need to be carefully tempered to allow the patient to adapt to his newly acquired circumstances.

Heart surgery

Patients undergoing coronary artery surgery require special consideration. To alleviate pre-operative and post-operative anxiety, the nature, indications and risks of the procedure should be explained. The patients should also be informed of the surroundings and the interventions they may expect when they arrive back from surgery into intensive care. Surgical patients are particularly prone to recurrent anxiety and depression after recovery, and therefore to poor rehabilitation results, because of persistent symptoms associated with the chest and leg incisions. They require explanation about the non-cardiac nature of symptoms arising from the chest wall, their normal persistence for weeks or months, and the integrity and rapid and complete healing of all the structures involved in surgery. Except in exceptional circumstances, most surgical patients should be advised about the physical and psychological benefits of early ambulation and discharge from hospital, and an early resumption of a normal life.

PERSONALITY AND STRESS

Type A behaviour, defined as the aggressive, time-conscious, ambitious, entrepreneurial or workaholic type, has been classified as a risk for coronary heart disease. According to some authors, it is an independent predictor of a propensity to myocardial infarction and other manifestations of coronary disease. First described by Friedman and Rosenman in 1956 (Friedman & Rosenman 1974) and still the subject of investigation and controversy, the concept of type A behaviour has not received widespread support from cardiologists despite the imprimatur of some official bodies and expert committees. The role of type A behaviour in coronary heart disease has been fully reviewed (Review Panel on Coronary-Prone Behaviour 1981).

Whether the propensity to coronary heart disease noted in type A individuals is independent of confounding factors, such as smoking, hypertension and hyperlipidaemia, is difficult to decide, but, from the practical point of achieving satisfactory results from our rehabilitation endeavours, it is wise to identify type A behaviour and to encourage a modification of such behaviour through appropriate counselling. Successful modification of type A behaviour can be achieved and is desirable if only to improve the patient's quality of life. Such modification may play a part in improving compliance to desirable behavioural changes, including control of smoking and alcohol abuse, and better attention to dieting and exercise guidelines. There are reports of a reduced incidence of fresh coronary events in patients subjected to type A modification (Review Panel on Coronary-Prone Behaviour 1981), but the prospect of improving quality of life also justifies appropriate counselling in these patients.

STRESS AND CORONARY HEART DISEASE

Stress in the public mind, and to a certain extent in the professional mind, is perceived as a key factor in causing coronary disease and in precipitating a heart attack. Apart from much circumstantial evidence linking two common events (a stressful event or stressful circumstances, often perceived retrospectively, and one of the acute manifestations of coronary heart disease), there is little basis for the popular view of stress as a cause of coronary heart disease, whatever its role in precipitating ischaemia or arrhythmias. For instance, there is some evidence that episodes of symptomatic or silent ischaemia can be precipitated by acute stressful situations, and that life-threatening arrhythmias can be provoked by emotional reactions in high risk cases.

In the course of counselling, we should seek stressful influences and circumstances which we consider to be a source of distress and concern to our patients. Such intervention can be productive in terms of quality of life and behaviour modification. At the same time, it is reassuring to the patient if we emphasise that some stress is normal in our lives, that it will not increase the risk of further infarction or sudden death, and that we have physiological mechanisms to cope with day-to-day stressful events.

Some patients confirm that their sense of well-being and enjoyment of life has improved since their heart attack. This satisfactory result of rehabilitation measures can often be attributed to life-style changes such as cessation of smoking and adoption of exercise programmes, but the perceived benefits of rehabilitation are not infrequently attributed to improved attitudes and better adaptation as a result of stress modification and counselling.

FAMILY AND SOCIAL SUPPORT

The patient who survives a myocardial infarction or who has recovered from heart surgery is faced with a number of obstacles to overcome in the course of returning to a normal life. These include the psychological impact of the illness or operation, including the loss of self-esteem and self-control. Patients almost invariably need to make major and permanent changes in life-style, such as adopting an exercise programme, stopping smoking and following certain dietary guidelines. Longterm medication and regular medical supervision may also be necessary. All these obstacles can be overcome, particularly if the patient receives the necessary guidelines and support from the medical team. The process of adaptation is considerably facilitated if family and friends can be actively supportive of the patient during the recovery stage. Support implies creating a milieu of encouragement and understanding which implicitly assumes that the patient is capable of returning to a normal life, and which eschews the cautious and overprotective role which family members were too often inclined to adopt in the past, largely as a result of the profession's very restrictive past attitudes to the management of coronary heart disease.

Support can also be effectively provided for the patient who needs to change life habits. The dietary needs of the patient can quite readily and usefully be adopted by the whole family as part of a policy of good nutrition. Smoking in the home of the ex-smoking patient should be discouraged, at least in the early stages of cessation, but, best of all, other members of the family can help the patient and themselves by eschewing the habit. The family can also join in the patient's exercise programme, thus making exercise more enjoyable and contributing to good family morale.

Unnecessary reference to the patient's illness should be avoided but family members should be aware of the need to identify significant symptoms and particularly any complaint of fresh cardiac pain, either at rest or with less exercise than usual. Under these circumstances, it is important to seek a medical opinion. Some physicians and rehabilitation centres recommend family training in cardio-pulmonary resuscitation in the high risk patients, such as those with a history of arrhythmias or recurring unstable angina. This recommendation seems sensible, assuming that problems of anxiety can be avoided.

The support of friends and fellow employees, 'buddy' support as described in the United States, is also desirable but less easy to arrange. The patients themselves can frequently outline the support they need from their friends, particularly in relation to life-style changes. Like family members, friends and colleagues should not adopt an advisory role. They should not refer excessively to the patient's illness nor, indeed, should patients seek advice from lay people. One not infrequently meets patients who become discouraged and depressed because of spurious advice received from or comments made by untutored lay people. Patients should be advised to avoid discussing their illness because of the mistaken significance they may attach to well intentioned but erroneous advice, and because it retards their recovery from a sick role position.

At least one responsible family member should be kept informed of the nature and management of the patient's illness from the time of admission to hospital. Attendance by the spouse and other family members at group educational and exercise sessions is desirable and is now often the rule.

Family members can be encouraged to adopt a more supportive role by seeking routine screening for coronary risk factors, and by seeking advice about their own life-styles. A coronary illness in a family is an appropriate time to encourage a primary prevention approach to heart illness and an opportunity of assisting people to take responsibility for their own and their families' health. In certain countries, coronary patients have formed self-supporting groups or 'coronary clubs' (Konig 1978, Wenger 1981). These organisations have proved most successful in helping patients and their families to understand the nature of coronary disease and take an active part in management and secondary prevention. These groups have also given an opportunity to well motivated medical practitioners to encourage a positive approach to health and prevention, and they have indirectly helped to educate the medical profession in this important aspect of medical care.

REFERENCES

Conroy R, Mulcahy R 1989 Psychological factors in cardiac rehabilitation. The Practitioner 233:748-752

Conroy R M, McGowan, E, Mulcahy R 1989 Improved subjective health in patients in a post-coronary rehabilitation programme. Irish Journal of Psychological Medicine 6:30-34

Friedman M, Rosenman R H 1974 Type A behaviour and your heart. A Knopf, New York

Guiry R M, Conroy R M, Hickey N, Mulcahy R 1987 Psychological response to an acute coronary event and its effect on subsequent rehabilitation and lifestyle change. Clinical Cardiology 10:256-260

Konig K 1978 Organization of rehabilitation centres. Advances in Cardiology 24:136-145

Review Panel on Coronary-Prone Behaviour and Coronary Heart Disease 1981. Coronary-prone behaviour and coronary heart disease: a critical review. Circulation 63:119-215

Stern T A 1987 Psychiatric management of acute myocardial infarction in the coronary care unit. American Journal of Cardiology 60:J59-67

Wenger N K 1981 Rehabilitation in 'Coronary Clubs'. In: Konig K (ed) Progress in echocardiography and radionuclide methods. Lifelong rehabilitation in phase III. Waldrick, Frieburg, pp 91-93

FURTHER READING

Birdwood G F B (ed) 1987 Quality of life—how it can be assessed and improved. Ciba-Geigy, Basle

16. Rehabilitation following coronary and valve surgery and cardiac transplantation

REHABILITATION AFTER CORONARY ARTERY SURGERY

The principles governing rehabilitation after myocardial infarction apply equally to patients submitted to coronary artery by-pass surgery. However, surgical patients do require special attention to specific problems arising out of the procedure. It is imperative that they should have a clear understanding of the purpose and nature of surgery beforehand, and that they should be forewarned of the various intensive care procedures. They also need to be reassured subsequently about the various symptoms which arise following a thoracotomy. These symptoms may persist for some months after surgery and may be perceived by the patient as being of cardiac origin. Full and repeated explanation and reassurance may be required to alleviate such anxiety.

Because surgery usually achieves considerable symptomatic relief in anginal patients, and is frequently perceived to be a life-saving measure by the patient, a rapid recovery and restoration to a normal life and to normal activities should be the rule. However, a return to a normal life, in terms of a return to work and the adoption of exercise programmes, has been less than satisfactory among surgical patients. These disappointing rehabilitation results may be attributed to a number of causes, including anxiety induced by the thoracotomy procedure and by the post-operative symptoms, inadequate rehabilitation attention on the part of the patient's medical advisors, a prolonged period of invalidism before operation, and an overcautious approach to the patient's capabilities on the part of the spouse, family members, and the family doctor.

These and other factors regarding rehabilitation should be sought and steps should be taken to counsel the patient and relatives about the favourable prospects of returning to a completely normal life provided by successful revascularisation. Prolonged hospitalisation and convalescence should be avoided, a prompt return to a normal life should be encouraged, and an active exercise programme should be designed to suit the patient's circumstances, preferences, and capabilities. It is also imperative that the patient, family members and family doctor should be aware of the vulnerability of the grafts and the native coronary vessels to progress of atherosclerosis in the presence of persistent coronary risk factors. Smoking and blood pressure control, and strict control of hyperlipidaemia, are essential, not only to reduce the risk of progression of arterial diseases but also to increase the patient's confidence in his or her future health and quality of life.

It is likely that smoking following coronary artery surgery is a factor in graft disease and occlusion, progression of atherosclerosis in the native vessels, and recurrence of angina and fresh myocardial infarction. Hyperlipidaemia has also been identified as a cause of post-operative deterioration (Campeau et al 1984). If the lipid profile of anginal patients cannot be normalised by dietary means, we should not hesitate to prescribe an appropriate lipid-lowering drug or combination of drugs. The modern pharmacology of hyperlipidaemia should make the normalisation of the lipid profile a feasible objective in all patients, except in the most severe homozygous cases.

There is little doubt that attention to the special rehabilitation needs of post-surgical patients will greatly improve their prospects of a successful return to a normal life, to a better quality of life, and probably an improved life expectation.

ANGIOPLASTY

Patients undergoing angioplasty require routine rehabilitation advice and supervision. However, there has been a high incidence of recurrence of symptoms and delayed myocardial infarction in those who are deemed to have benefited from angioplasty (Baim 1988). Such patients require careful and regular supervision following the procedure. They should be advised beforehand about the risks of precipitating an acute ischaemic or infarct event, and about the possible need for emergency revascularisation.

REHABILITATION AFTER VALVE SURGERY

The principles of rehabilitation recommended in patients after myocardial infarction or coronary artery surgery—early return to a normal life in social, recreational, vocational and psychological terms, combined with reduction of complications and risk of further events, and with a good quality of life—apply also to patients following valve surgery. In non-coronary surgical cases, however, special circumstances may exist which require emphasis.

Many patients undergoing surgery for mitral or aortic valve disease may have been partially or completely invalided for a considerable length of time before operation. These patients may have had a prolonged period off work or, indeed, may never have had training for or experience of work. Their chronic progressive disability may have made them dependent on others, both medically and psychologically. These circumstances create special problems in relation to the resumption of a normal independent life after successful surgery, and may be a serious, even intractable, impediment to such an outcome. A close correlation has been reported between the length of pre-operative disability and poor return to work rates after all forms of heart surgery. A number of factors may play a part in determining this correlation but an important factor is an impairment of motivation, initiative, and self-esteem created by a long period of dependency. This dependency is frequently unrelated to the degree of functional recovery following surgery.

Achieving a normal vocational, social and psychological recovery in patients following valve surgery requires careful pre- and post-operative counselling. It requires the intervention of a dedicated social worker and occupational therapist, as well as physician and surgeon. Family attitudes can play a major role in discouraging satisfactory rehabilitation, when the patient's invalid role may have become an integral part of family life, a circumstance which may be difficult to change. The relatives themselves may be reluctant to accept a new role for the patient. The advice and co-operation of the family must, therefore, be harnessed. The objects of the operation, including its aim in improving the patient's functional capacity, should be explained beforehand to the family as well as the patient.

Longterm medical supervision and medication, such as anticoagulant therapy, may be required in post-surgical patients. This may create an impediment when encouraging an independent attitude on the part of the patient, but continued medical supervision and treatment should not prejudice a satisfactory return to normal and to an independent existence if the purpose of treatment is understood and normal activities are encouraged. It should be made clear that there are other benefits derived from successful surgery, as well as reducing complications and improving longevity.

REHABILITATION AFTER HEART TRANSPLANTATION

Cardiac transplantation patients invariably continue to be supervised and cared for by the specialist transplantation team. Many recipients will have been invalided for a considerable length of time before transplantation, thus making a return to a normal independent life, and a return to work, more difficult but not by any means impossible to achieve. Transplant patients, because they are younger and have unique post-operative problems, require special attention to achieve good rehabilitation results.

Survival rates following transplantation continue to improve, particularly since the advent of cyclosporin in controlling the major hazard of organ rejection. The International Society for Heart Transplantation reported on the outcome in 3623 heart transplant operations performed during the preceding five years (Kaye 1987). There was an 81% one-year survival and a 78% five-year survival.

Teams caring for transplant patients have been particularly assiduous, not only in dealing with rejection problems and other causes of post-operative morbidity and mortality, but also in encouraging patients to return to a normal physical and psychosocial life. Improved quality of life is an integral part of an improved psychosocial life, and should invariably be achieved in patients who, in general, have been severely disabled before surgery. In earlier reports return to work rates have been variable, but it is clear from present experience that satisfactory return to work rates and satisfactory psychosocial adjustment can be achieved (Worcester 1988). Mood changes, such as anxiety, can occur after operation, and these changes need to be anticipated and treated. Careful pre-operative counselling plays an important part in the patient's subsequent psychosocial adjustment. Patients may be particularly concerned about graft rejection, the need for longterm medication, and by personal and economic factors affecting themselves and their families.

Personal difficulties may include loss of libido and impotence, which may contribute to marital discord. Appropriate counselling of both patient and spouse should be helpful in achieving satisfactory sexual adjustment. As in patients recovering from myocardial infarction or coronary artery surgery, patients and spouses may be reluctant to broach the question of sexual maladjustment, and therefore should be encouraged to raise the issue, if it proves to be relevant. In this area, and in dealing with the wider issues of rehabilitation, family and social support is mandatory, so that the spouse and family members should have a thorough understanding of the rationale of the operation and of post-operative management.

Post-operative psychological changes, such as anxiety and depression, may be concealed by denial, which is reported to be commonplace in cardiac transplant patients (Mai 1986). Denial may, if severe, interfere with the patient's motivation to adhere strictly to medication and to other behavioural guidelines. Counselling and adequate longterm supervision by the rehabilitation team should suffice to control the most extreme effects of denial.

Rehabilitation practices after transplantation have been more thorough and more clearly defined than practices after myocardial infarction and coronary artery surgery. This almost certainly has to do with problems of rejection and with the major psychological adjustments which are common to the transplant patients. It also has to do with the effect that careful supervision exerts on post-operative morbidity and mortality. Without good and sustained rehabilitation practices, cardiac transplantation would fall into disrepute. At least to some extent, any disrepute which may be associated with post-myocardial infarction and post-coronary artery surgery management may be attributed to our relative neglect of longterm management needs.

The practical and psychosocial aspects of cardiac transplantation have been well reviewed by Marion Worcester (1988).

REFERENCES

Baim D S 1988 In: E Braunwald (ed) Heart disease: a text book of cardiovascular medicine (3rd edition). W B Saunders and Co, Philadephia, pp 1379-1389

Campeau L, Enjalbert M. Lesperance J et al 1984 The relation of risk factors to the development of atherosclerosis in saphenous-vein bypass grafts and the progression of disease in the native circulation. A study 10 years after aortocoronary bypass surgery. New England Journal of Medicine 311:1329-1332

Kaye M P 1987 The Registry of the International Society for Heart Transplantation: fourth official report 1987. Journal of Heart Transplantation 6:63-67

Mai F M 1986 Graft and donor denial in heart transplant recipients. American Journal of Psychiatry 143:1159-1161

Worcester M C 1988 Psychosocial aspects of cardiac transplantation (editorial). Medical Journal of Australia 149:115-116

Index